A Patient-Centered Approach to Optimizing Ambulatory Access:

Insights From Leaders in Academic Medicine

ASSOCIATION OF AMERICAN MEDICAL COLLEGES
WASHINGTON, D.C.

VIZIENT
IRVING, TEXAS

AUTHORS

Danielle Carder, MSc; Nicole Spatafora, MS-HSM; Scott Shipman, MD, MPH; Marilyn Sherrill, RN, MBA; Robert Dean, DO, MBA

ABOUT US

AAMC

The AAMC (Association of American Medical Colleges) is a not-for-profit association dedicated to transforming health through medical education, health care, medical research, and community collaborations. Its members are all 155 accredited U.S. and 17 accredited Canadian medical schools; more than 400 teaching hospitals and health systems, including Department of Veterans Affairs medical centers; and more than 70 academic societies. Through these institutions and organizations, the AAMC leads and serves America's medical schools and teaching hospitals and their more than 179,000 full-time faculty members, 92,000 medical students, 140,000 resident physicians, and 60,000 graduate students and postdoctoral researchers in the biomedical sciences. Additional information about the AAMC is available at aamc.org.

Vizient

Vizient, Inc., provides solutions and services that improve the delivery of high-value care by aligning cost, quality, and market performance for more than 50% of the nation's acute-care providers, which includes 97% of the nation's academic medical centers, and more than 20% of ambulatory providers. Vizient provides expertise, analytics, and advisory services, as well as a contract portfolio that represents more than $100 billion in annual purchasing volume, to improve patient outcomes and lower costs. Vizient has earned a World's Most Ethical Company designation from the Ethisphere Institute every year since its inception. Headquartered in Irving, Texas, Vizient has offices throughout the United States. Learn more at vizientinc.com.

Clinical Practice Solutions Center

Based upon more than 20 years of collaboration between the AAMC and Vizient, the Clinical Practice Solutions Center (CPSC) creates one solution for medical practices of all sizes. With guided analytics, medical practice leaders can examine their own data related to provider productivity, coding, revenue, and charge capture as well as patient access. Together with benchmarking data, the CPSC puts the power of data into the hands of academic medical centers and community practice organizations just like yours. With the ability to examine data at the department, specialty, and provider levels, the CPSC allows for easy comparisons across key performance indicators. Using comparative data, advisory support, and peer collaboration, the CPSC is an essential component of every clinical practice leader's tool kit. Learn more at clinicalpracticesolutionscenter.org.

Suggested citation: AAMC, Vizient. *A Patient-Centered Approach to Optimizing Ambulatory Access: Insights From Leaders in Academic Medicine*. Washington, DC: AAMC and Vizient; 2021.

ISBN: 978-1-57754-200-1

CONTENTS

EXECUTIVE SUMMARY

Facilitating access to care for patients is focused on ensuring timely, necessary, and appropriate health care services. Improving access to care is a strategic priority for most academic health systems and a challenge for nearly all. To support systems in meeting that challenge, the AAMC and Vizient sought insights from ambulatory care leaders, physicians, and staff in academic medical centers (AMCs) whose organizations' access performance has been exemplary. A standard method was used to select the organizations from participants in the AAMC-Vizient Clinical Practice Solutions Center (CPSC) that submit data to the Vizient Ambulatory Quality and Accountability (AQA) Scorecard. Five academic health systems ranking in the top 10 for the AQA Access domain from 2016 to 2018 were identified for study. In-person site visits with executive leaders, clinical leaders, and frontline providers were conducted to better understand the strengths, opportunities, effectiveness, and efficiency of access operations. **Five organizations** contributed to this work:

- Emory Healthcare
- Harborview Medical Center
- NYU Langone Faculty Group Practice
- Stanford Health Care
- University of Colorado Hospital

A **framework** was developed based on common themes from the visits and calls with these high-performing organizations. The primary drivers behind patient-centered access to care, listed below, are supported in the report by secondary drivers and examples. While some examples are unique to a single organization and others are common, any organization can use them to support their own access strategy.

- **ENGAGED LEADERSHIP:** High-performing organizations have leaders who provide vision and unwavering commitment to achieving strategic goals tied to improved access.
- **STRUCTURE AND STANDARD PROCESSES:** An access strategy is more apt to succeed if it is structured and uses standard processes that reduce unwarranted variation and lead to improved access to care.
- **ACTIONABLE DATA AND ANALYTICS:** Ensuring data validity and conducting thoughtful analysis to determine the underlying story informs the critical steps in improving access.
- **OPTIMIZE CARE DELIVERY:** Optimizing care delivery and the care team is crucial to maximizing capacity and increasing throughput (the number of patients seen per clinic session) while providing high-quality care. Evaluating the types of care and services provided is essential to understanding the mix of staff needed to deliver care and improve access.
- **WORKFORCE ENGAGEMENT:** Plans for engaging the workforce are designed to reduce turnover, build skills, foster community, and create alignment with organizational access goals.
- **LEVERAGE TECHNOLOGY:** Technology must be leveraged to meet patients' demands for convenience, quality, and timeliness of access. Meeting patients where they are is an important access strategy.

This report focuses on health system-based efforts to enhance timely and appropriate access to care in the ambulatory clinic setting. Leaders can use the framework for action and examples from several leading academic health systems as they work on ways to improve access.

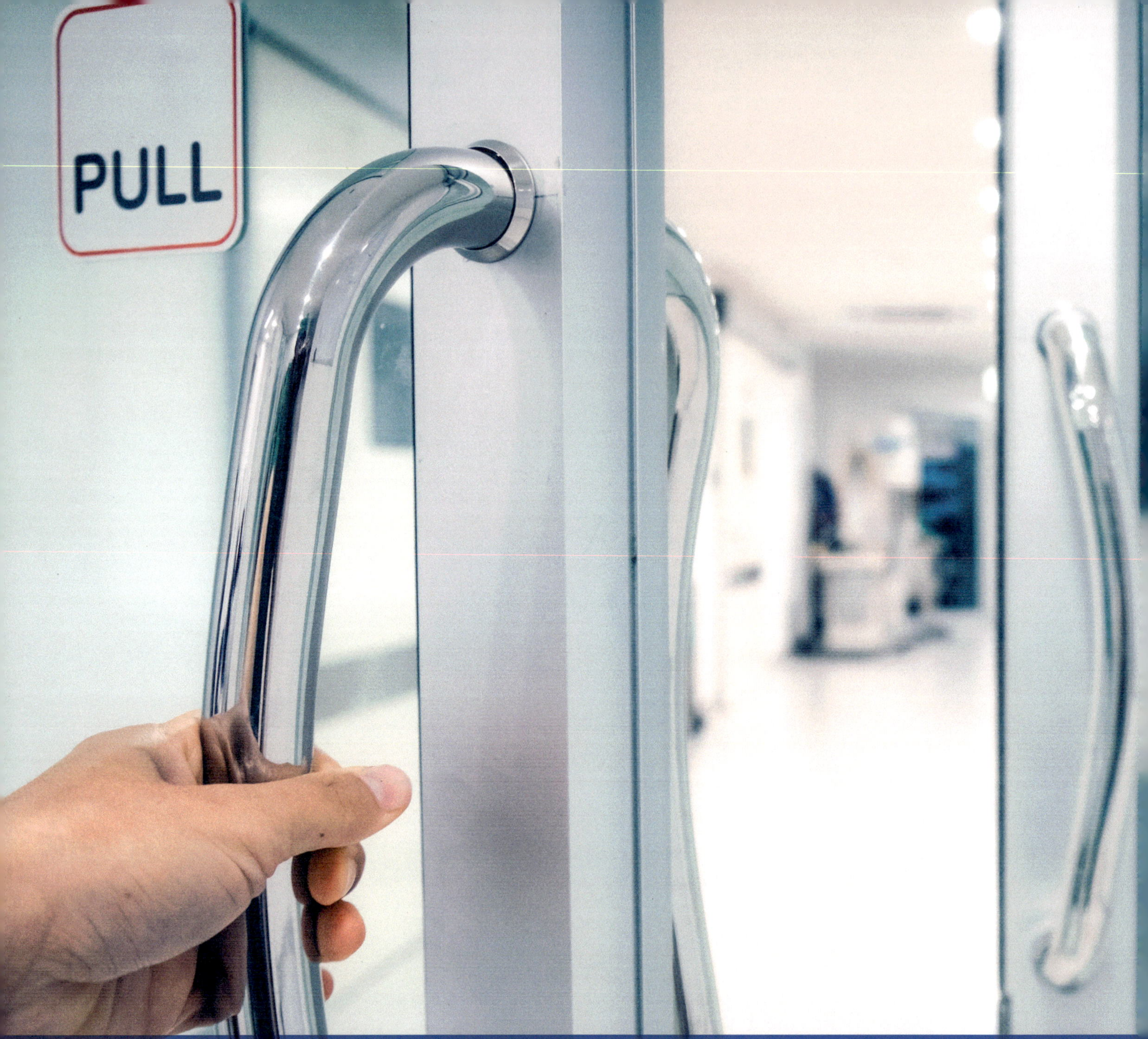

Introduction

Facilitating patients' access to health care involves helping people acquire the necessary and appropriate health care resources to overcome the numerous barriers to access. Access to health care, as defined by the National Academy of Medicine, is "the timely use of personal health services to achieve the best health outcomes."[1] Equally important to timely care is having the right care in the right setting.

According to the U.S. Census, the U.S. population is projected to increase more than 19% between 2017 and 2060, from about 326 million to 404 million, with people aged 65 and older growing from 15% to 25% of the population.[2] As the population ages and demand for care increases, concerns about physician workforce shortages are growing. The AAMC predicts estimated shortages will continue for physician providers, and by 2033, there will be an estimated shortage of 21,400-55,200 primary care physicians and 33,700-86,700 non-primary care specialists.[3] These changes are creating challenges and barriers that can lead to longer wait times and difficulty accessing care. According to data from the Clinical Practice Solutions Center (CPSC), the median wait time for new-patient visits in 2019 ranged from nine to 38 days across medical and surgical specialties.[4] In a study by National Public Radio, the Robert Wood Johnson Foundation, and the Harvard T.H. Chan School of Public Health, about one in five patients (22%) said there was at least one time in the past two years when they needed health care but could not see their regular provider.[5] Among the patients who could not see their regular provider, 52% said it was because either their doctor did not have any available appointment times or their doctor was away from the office.These reports and others have shown that the limited capacity to meet the growing demand strains most academic health systems today.

Health insurance coverage and the quality and completeness of the terms of that coverage are highly politicized and hotly debated subjects in society. As critical as insurance coverage is to facilitating access, coverage alone does not ensure it. This report focuses on health system-based efforts to enhance timely and appropriate access to care in the ambulatory clinic setting. It presents a framework for action and examples from several leading academic health systems from across the country for leaders to consider as they improve access for their patient populations.

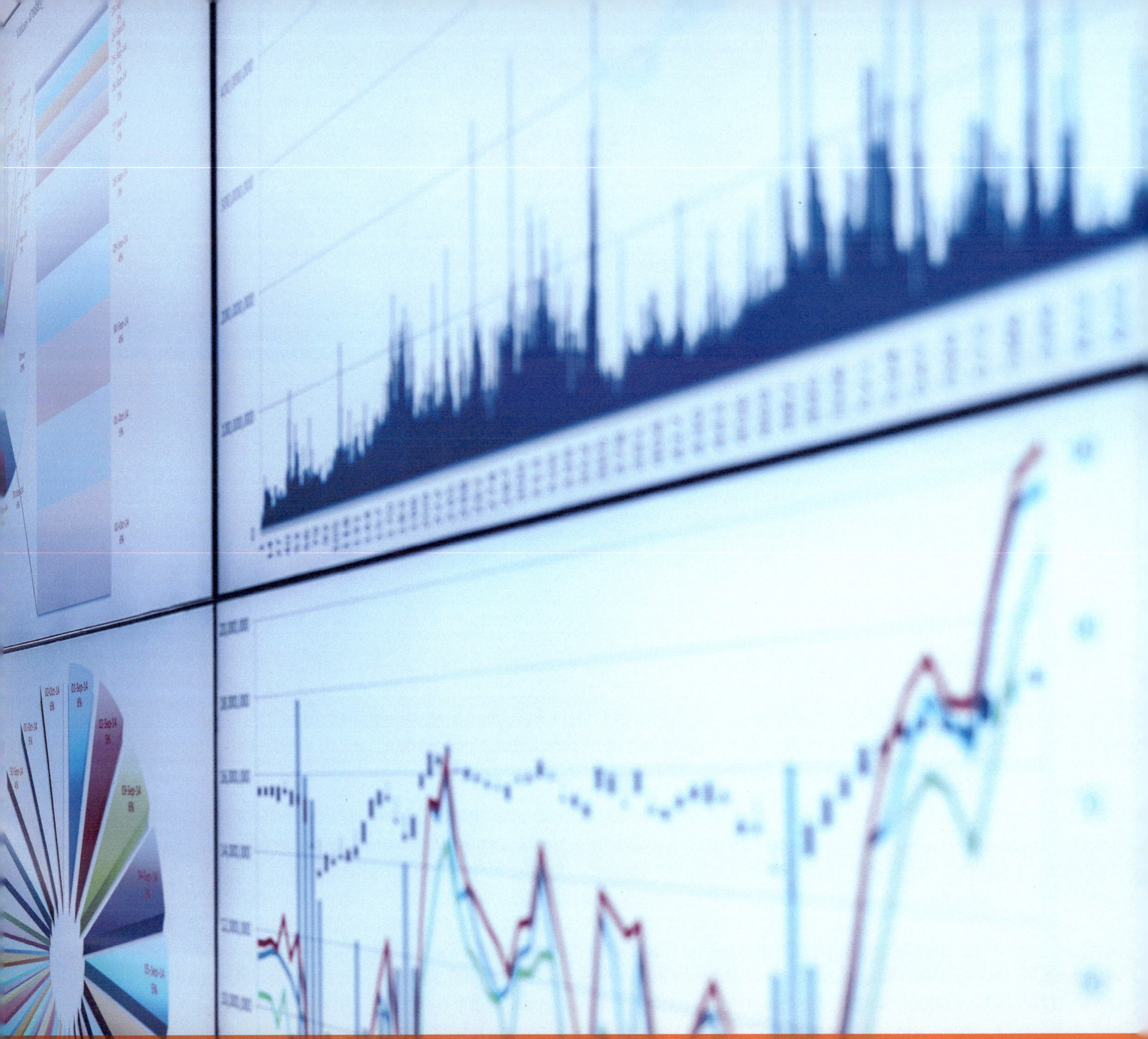

Method Used to Select Exemplar Organizations

The AAMC and Vizient established the Access Initiative in 2018, beginning with the publication of *Learning and Leading in Access to Care: An Overview of Member Collaboratives.*[6] The purpose of this study was to develop a deeper understanding of the innovations and effective strategies ambulatory care leaders, physicians, and staff in academic medical centers (AMCs) are using to improve patient access. The search for critical success factors and barriers to access associated with these efforts led to the following questions:

- **What effective approaches and practices to enhancing patient access are used today?**
- **How is access evaluated and measured in organizations focused on access?**
- **What are the most promising levers for improvement and change?**

To answer these questions, the AAMC and Vizient looked for exemplary performers that participate in the AAMC-Vizient CPSC and submit data to the Vizient Ambulatory Quality and Accountability (AQA) scorecard. Academic medical systems consistently ranking in the top 10 for the AQA Access domain in the three-year period were identified as exemplary. The Access domain includes the following CPSC measures, based on data from the second quarter of 2015 through the first quarter of 2018 for 17 specialties measured in the AQA scorecard.[7]

- **Appointments Canceled by Provider or Clinic (Bumped) Within 30 days of Appointment Date (% of total appointments).**
- **New Patients Seen Within 10 days of Scheduling Appointment (%).**
- **New-Patient Median Lag (days between scheduling and patients being seen).**
- **New-Patient Visits (% of total visits).**
- **No-Show Appointments or Same- or Previous-Day Cancellations Preceding Appointment (%).**

Seven organizations that consistently ranked at the top among peers or had significant improvements in this domain between 2015 and 2018 were selected for further study. Semi-structured phone interviews building from the same questions were conducted with contacts at each organization. From these phone interviews, five member organizations were selected for in-person site visits. Single-day, in-person site meetings between October and December 2019 consisted of discussions with executive leaders, clinical leaders, and care providers to better understand the strengths, opportunities, effectiveness, and efficiency of their health care-access operations. Information from the site visits was synthesized into an access framework, and contacts at each organization reviewed and validated the site findings before publication.

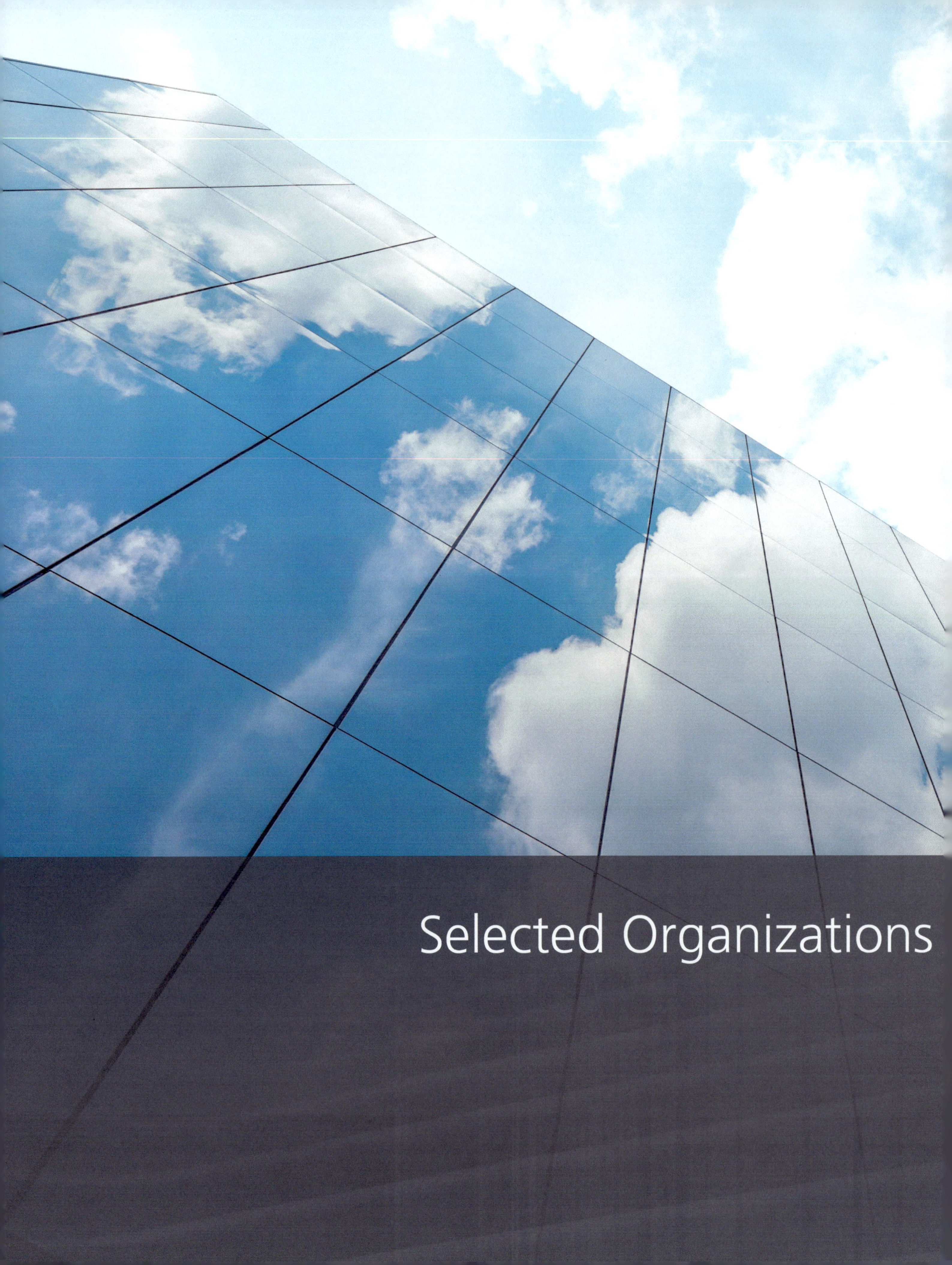

Selected Organizations

Emory Healthcare (Emory) is the most comprehensive health system in Georgia, with net revenues of $4.7 billion annually, 11 hospitals, more than 250 locations, and 5 million annual outpatient visits. Emory Healthcare employs more than 33,000 staff and has about 2,800 physicians and 1,000 advanced practice providers (APPs) who practice across more than 70 medical specialties.

Harborview Medical Center (Harborview) is owned by the citizens of King County, governed by a board of trustees appointed by King County, and managed by the University of Washington (UW). There are eight entities in the UW Medicine health system, with clinics associated with multiple hospitals representing more than 2,000 physicians and health care professionals. As the only Level I Adult and Pediatric Trauma Center in Washington, Harborview Medical Center provides specialized comprehensive emergency services to patients throughout the region and serves as the disaster preparedness and disaster control hospital for King County, including Seattle. Clinic visits to Harborview total more than 300,000 annually.

NYU Langone Faculty Group Practice (NYU) has undergone tremendous growth and expansion over the past 10 years. Beginning with practices located in a "super block" in Manhattan, the faculty practice has grown to include about 350 locations across Manhattan, Brooklyn, Queens, and Long Island and more than 7.85 million ambulatory visits annually. From 2011 to 2019, the number of physicians employed by the NYU Grossman School of Medicine grew from 845 to more than 3,200. The faculty practice's strategy is to build out primary care to support growth in specialty care.

Stanford Health Care (SHC) is a large academic health system headquartered in Palo Alto (Calif.) with about 200 clinics in more than 50 locations throughout the Bay Area. SHC includes more than 3,000 clinically active physicians, including about 350 community providers and 2,500 faculty from the Stanford University School of Medicine. Of the 350 community providers, about 250 are primary care providers (PCPs). Conversely, the faculty is composed of specialists and about 75 PCPs.

University of Colorado Hospital (Colorado), a founding hospital of the UCHealth system, and University of Colorado School of Medicine are centered in the Denver market on the Anschutz Medical Campus (AMC). The AMC is the only academic medical center in Colorado, which has experienced considerable population growth recently. The 12 hospitals in the UCHealth system have 5,000 affiliated or employed physicians. Last year, the hospitals served nearly 600,000 unique patients across the clinical settings in Colorado, with 4.5 million outpatient, urgent-care, and emergency room visits. The University of Colorado School of Medicine is also a regional center for many pediatric and adult specialties, drawing patients from across the Rocky Mountain region.

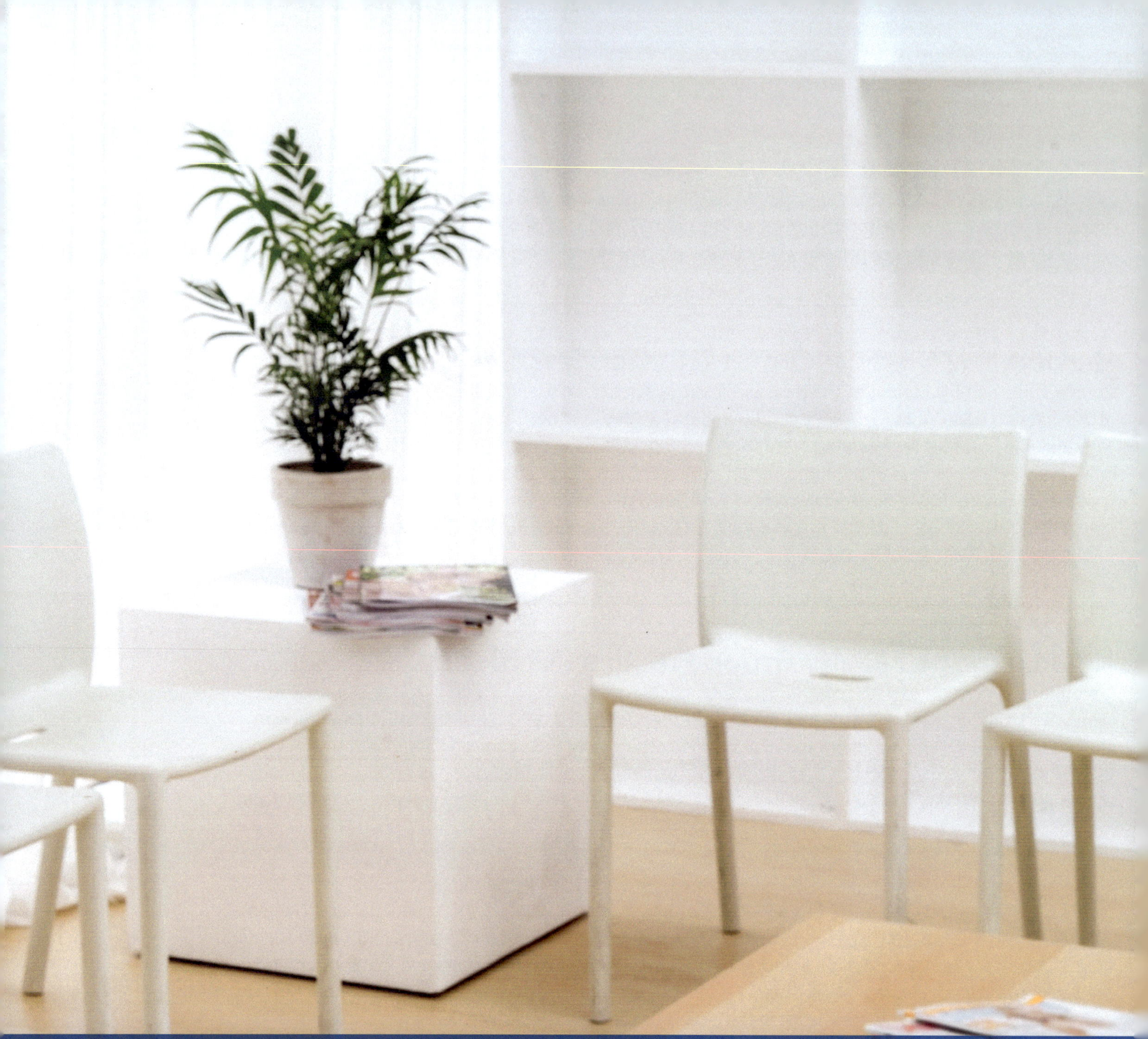

Framework for Optimizing Access to Care in the Ambulatory Setting

An access framework was developed based on common themes from the site visits and telephone calls with the five high-performing organizations (Figure 1). The framework demonstrates the relationship between the overall aim of the project — to optimize patient-centered access to ambulatory care — and the primary and secondary drivers that help achieve this aim. The five organizations highlighted in this report exemplified the primary and secondary drivers included in the access framework. This report includes real-life examples of these primary and secondary drivers. The access framework, drivers, and examples provide leading strategies any organization could use to support its access strategy.

INITIATE

ENGAGED LEADERSHIP

- System growth and access strategy
- Access governance and leadership structure
- Culture

DEVELOP

STRUCTURE AND STANDARD PROCESSES

- Scheduling
- Capacity and demand management
- Systemwide policies and work processes
- Data-driven performance improvement

ACTIONABLE DATA AND ANALYTICS

- Metric selection and measurement
- Data integrity
- Data reporting and transparency

ENABLE

OPTIMIZE CARE DELIVERY

- Team-based care
- Population health management
- Performance optimization
- Equitable, patient-centered care

WORKFORCE ENGAGEMENT

- Onboarding
- Education and training
- Incentives, recognition, and rewards

LEVERAGE TECHNOLOGY

- Electronic medical record optimization
- Virtual health capabilities
- Digital front door
- Artificial intelligence and predictive analytics

Figure 1. Framework for optimizing ambulatory access to care. (Select any icon for more information.)

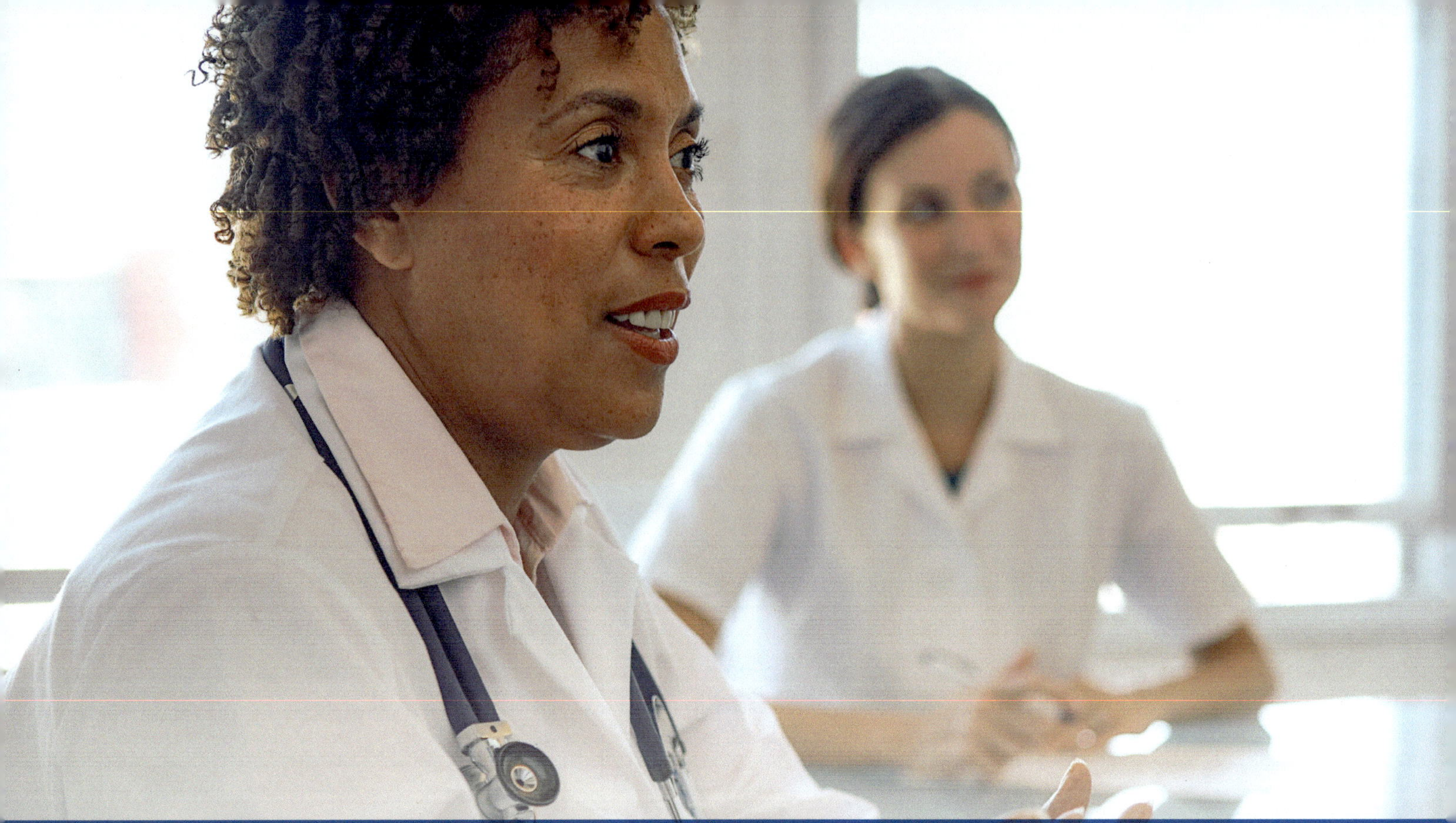

Primary Driver: Engaged Leadership

High-performing organizations have leaders who provide vision and unwavering commitment to achieving strategic goals tied to improved access. These leaders recognize that continuous attention to detail is essential for sustaining improvements in access to care.

PRIMARY DRIVER	SECONDARY DRIVERS
Engaged Leadership	**System growth and access strategy:** Prioritize and develop an access strategy that informs a facility plan, a care-delivery model, how resources will be deployed, and the workforce needed to execute and deliver care.
	Access governance and leadership structure: Create a formalized leadership structure that includes the people responsible for specific access-related efforts and their oversight and governance, with clear lines of accountability at all levels of the organization.
	Culture: Ensure that access is ingrained in the organizational culture and is a focus within the organization and that all leaders, providers, administrators, and staff are moving toward a shared vision and goal.

AAMC vizient.

SYSTEM GROWTH AND ACCESS STRATEGY

Emory

Emory has focused on access as a core discipline since the early 2000s due to a board-directed initiative. Before then, patients were required to have a referral from a provider to gain access to an Emory provider. Although the referral requirement was removed in the 1990s, Emory leadership still works to dispel the misconception that a referral is required and has prioritized access as both a strategic and an operational priority within the organization. Emory Healthcare's most recent five-year strategic plan (which runs through 2024) includes access as a strategic priority area and best patient access and experience as a strategic goal. Emory has experienced exponential growth in the past three years through organic growth and merger-and-acquisition activity. To expand and diversify access, Emory has developed a geographically dispersed strategy and continues to execute local, regional, and national growth strategies. The CEO and chairman of the board of Emory Healthcare reinforces access as a strategic priority, conveying the idea to the physicians and clinician workforce that improved patient access is critical to the clinical mission of Emory University and, thus, to the educational and research missions.

Stanford Health Care

SHC's access journey began in 2008 with the strategic decision to expand beyond Palo Alto and Redwood City. The creation of the University Healthcare Alliance (UHA) in 2011 both established a foundation through which community physician clinics were supported and expanded SHC's geographic footprint. In 2014-2017, with enterprise-level strategic planning, the organization's governing objective shifted to creating value for patients, including improving the patient experience and quality of care, both of which involve improving access. A unique attribute of the SHC governance structure is the creation of a single set of priorities for both faculty and community clinicians through the Ambulatory Value Oversight Committee (AVOC). This committee reports to the Quality, Patient Safety and Effectiveness Committee and addresses all aspects of the value (V) equation: patient experience (E), access to care (S), quality of care (Q), and cost (C).

$$V = \left[\frac{Q + S}{C}\right] \times E$$

Stanford Health Care's Value Equation
Value of care equals quality of care plus access to care, divided by cost, times patient experience.

A unique feature of the SHC access strategy is the approach to employer contracts, which go beyond traditional payer relationships. For large organizations where access is essential, SHC determines whether an on-site clinic is needed. Alternatives to investing in an on-site clinic include providing on-site navigators. These individuals are trained in high-touch advocacy and interact with employees to help them navigate SHC services.

ACCESS GOVERNANCE AND LEADERSHIP STRUCTURE

NYU Langone

NYU Langone has a dyad leadership structure, that is, with both physician and executive oversight and governance of the faculty group practice. A supporting leadership structure of additional executives, called the executive team, is led by a vice president of ambulatory care operations and oversees the teams dedicated to ambulatory operations and ambulatory access. The ambulatory operations team, run by regional directors, oversees practice operations across multiple locations. The ambulatory access team oversees standardization and optimization of front-end operations, the access centers, digital access, workflow optimization, and training. NYU leadership sets and shares the access strategy and creates the standards and expectations, but it allows individual practices flexibility in how they implement this strategy. The bedrock of this approach is a commitment to oversight, quality assurance, and a centralized leadership infrastructure.

CULTURE

Harborview

Harborview is a mission-driven organization whose primary mission is to provide health care for the most vulnerable residents of King County. The organization's priority is to deliver care to these residents in the communities where they live by developing access points through specialized clinics and by expanding primary care services within the communities. The organization has adapted to meet the unique needs of vulnerable patients, including delivering care to patients where they live. The leadership emphasizes that everything Harborview does begins with the equity lens. What does that mean for this vulnerable population? What are the social determinants of health that could affect care delivery? The leadership focuses on population health management, developing services to meet unique patient needs, and engaging community partners in care delivery. Providers and staff at Harborview have internalized this mission-driven approach, recognizing patients' diverse needs (both medical and social) and helping patients address those needs in a variety of ways.

Colorado

Access has been a strategic priority for Colorado throughout the past eight years and was reinforced with the arrival of a new CEO who deemed access one of the organization's top five priorities. The Colorado culture centers around a pioneering mentality, collaboration among the provider groups, and a commitment to a patient-centered, team-based approach to care. Commitment to a performance-improvement mindset and practice transformation is also part of the culture. The organization's innovative spirit and commitment to technology inform the collaboration among the medical school, hospitals, and faculty practice. Nothing is done in isolation, including developing future growth strategies, care redesign, practice optimization, and focusing on measurement through common metrics. Being the only academic medical center in a growing market pushes the organization to innovate.

Leading Practices for Engaged Leadership

Engaged leadership with respect to access means leaders prioritize access — defining it as a pillar of the organization — and ensure a leadership team is accountable for access-operations performance. Consistent across the organizations with engaged leadership was a senior executive (typically, the chief medical officer) with direct oversight of access. Supporting this executive is a leadership structure with an identified administrative access leader (typically, vice president of access or higher) and a dedicated team responsible for access work. At each of these organizations, there was a clear culture change from the top down to recognize the importance of access and how it drives all other aspects of the organization's mission — from research to education. Cultural transformation is physician led and emphasizes the patient experience as the driver of change within the organization.

CHANGE TACTICS FOR ENGAGED LEADERSHIP

- ☑ Establish access as a foundational priority for your organization and incorporate access into your ambulatory care strategy.
- ☑ Create a formalized ambulatory care and access-to-care governance structure and leadership team with a dedicated leader who reports to the senior executive accountable for all access-related initiatives.
- ☑ Support the leadership structure with appropriate committees focused on access (e.g., patient experience and workflow optimization) so your organization includes the perspectives of additional stakeholders.
- ☑ Cultivate physician leaders at all levels within your organization who understand and are committed to having a strategy for increasing access to care and to executing that strategy.
- ☑ Set organizational access goals and directives but provide clinic and department leaders with operational flexibility to deliver results.
- ☑ Put the patient at the center to drive cultural change, which must be physician led to be successful, and engage patient and family advisors to help your organization prioritize access-improvement opportunities.

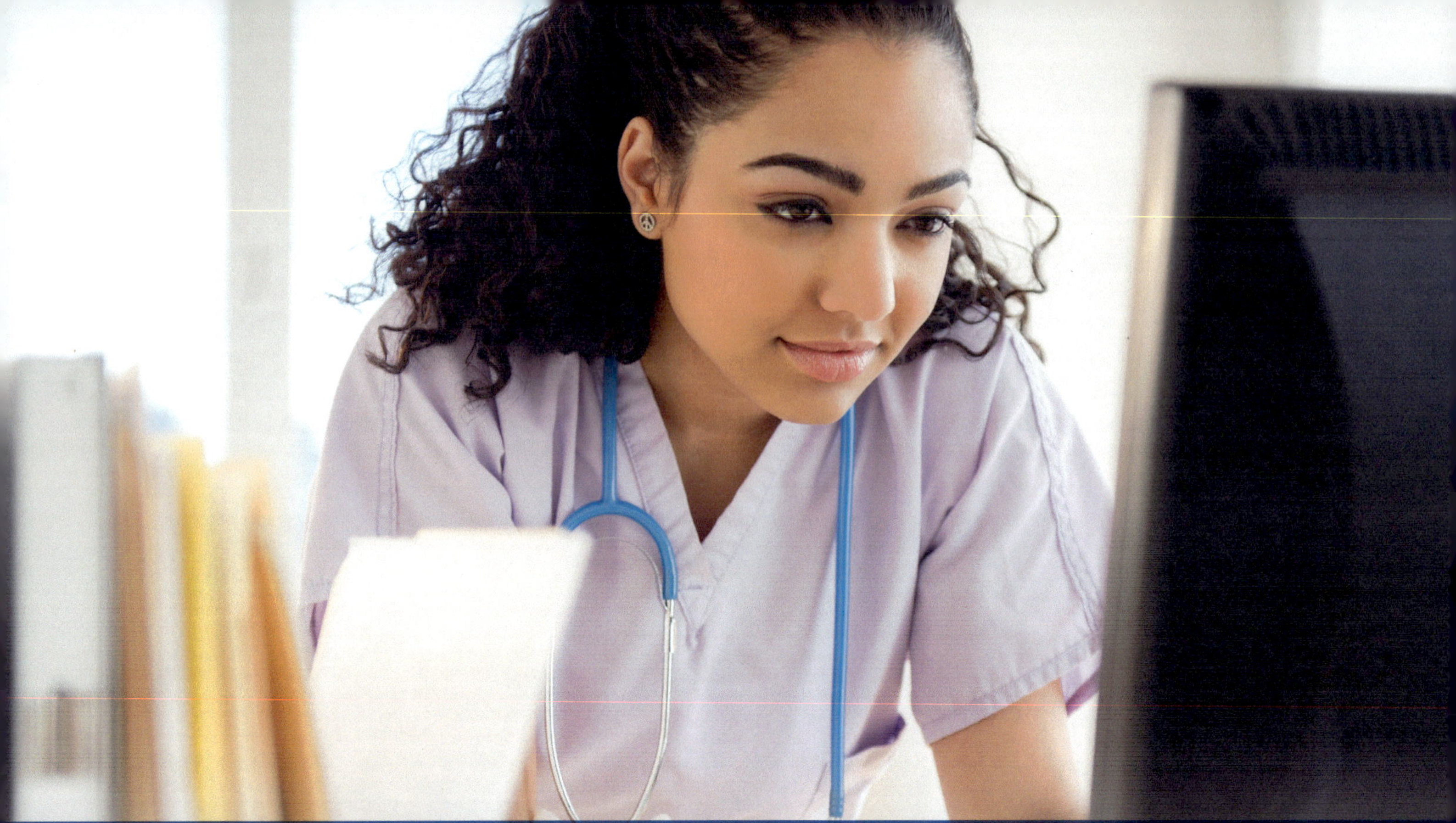

Primary Driver: Structure and Standard Processes

Successful implementation of an organizational access strategy benefits from a structure that includes standard processes to reduce unwarranted variation and improve access to care. Identifying the critical requirements and workflows and how these fit into the overall access strategy are key components of success.

PRIMARY DRIVER	SECONDARY DRIVERS
Structure and Standard Processes	**Scheduling:** Implement a centralized operation and scheduling system to remove silos and reduce variation and duplication that meets the needs of the organization and includes input from physicians and other key stakeholders.
	Capacity and demand management: Implement standard work processes and capacity-management strategies with a focus on appropriateness of care.
	Systemwide policies and work processes: Develop standardized, enterprise-wide policies related to scheduling clinics and appointments and related provider expectations.
	Data-driven performance improvement: Designate resources to support performance-improvement efforts, with a focus on driving change through data analytics and performance measurement.

SCHEDULING

Emory

Emory's centralized contact center began with primary care and expanded to some specialty clinics. Contact-center methodology with standardized tools, call-distribution capabilities, and call monitoring quickly became the recognized norm. Considerable time was needed to build specialty-specific expertise and to demonstrate how a patient-access team could help divisions achieve their access goals. Contact-center staff conduct field trips to clinics and in return, providers visit the contact center. The goal of these visits is to build relationships, allow contact-center staff to better understand the providers' practice, and allow provider teams to understand what frontline access colleagues are being asked to do. Today, the contact center answers calls for all 70 specialties across Emory's Physician Group Practices with a single team of agents and a leadership structure that oversees this centralized system. Significant investment has gone into workflow tools, online knowledge management, and call protocols that allow the team to provide high-level service across all clinical specialties. Access managers, in conjunction with their access colleagues, ensure clinical protocols, escalation pathways, and scheduling-related information are current. Each access manager uses standard forms, templates, and protocol development tools to ensure consistent information across all teams.

NYU

NYU has three stand-alone access centers across the continental United States. The centers' wide geographic distribution has provided patients with extended hours for scheduling appointments and increased capacity for answering calls and connecting with patients. With multiple locations aligned on the same technology, leadership of access centers can easily and reliably shift calls if challenges arise at a specific center. Visit types and template protocols are standardized across the access centers through the electronic medical record (EMR). Practices have reasonable flexibility to set visit durations and manage day-to-day details of their own provider templates. While there is flexibility, the corporate access team reviews templates and metrics to monitor compliance with standards, ensuring productivity targets and access goals are met.

The mantra for the access efforts at Colorado is "standardize what you can; customize what you have to."

Colorado

The mantra for the access efforts at Colorado is "standardize what you can; customize what you have to." Many providers resisted the creation of a centralized call center because they were worried about the clinics' losing control. The access team has five guiding principles for scheduling: standardize workflow to improve efficiency; reduce variability to reduce handling time; automate as much as possible to reduce call volume; require new practices requesting the centralized call center, Patient Line, to be proactively billed for its cost; and require newly onboarded practices to adapt to all existing workflows. The transition to centralized scheduling forced the system to become more structured and reduce variation in templates and visit types. Patient Line and practice staff and providers reviewed each practice to understand workflows and scheduling needs. Spreading out provider schedules across the day and week was one area of focus. These efforts toward centralizing and standardizing the use of decision trees in the EMR provided a more structured system while highlighting the need for variation and customization at each clinic — once again, embodying the principle of "standardize what you can; customize what you have to."

CAPACITY AND DEMAND MANAGEMENT

Emory

Emory has a centralized master scheduling and templating team that manages edits to all master and daily schedules. A critical step in centralizing was defining how long a clinic session or half-day was and standardizing this across specialties and providers. A single, dedicated team manages change requests against this master schedule. This team receives requests from specialty divisions through a ticketing system. The team includes capacity-management architects who evaluate the requested edits against key metrics such as relative value units (RVUs), budgets, ratios of new to returning patients, and provider capacity. The team guides the division on the potential impact of making the change. This team was critical to Emory's ability to achieve consistent performance in the top tier of Vizient's metrics for new-patient visits.

Emory also created a standard structure to better coordinate faculty hires. Department chairs, health system and Emory University School of Medicine leadership, and strategic planning team members meet to discuss strategic growth needs and faculty recruitment. This coordinated effort began with basic activities such as coordinating the hiring of additional surgeons with an assessment of need for compensatory growth in anesthesiologists. Department chairs and business managers determine where growth is needed. Ultimately, they assign a standardized, three-tier designation that indicates a department's ability to hire:

- Open: Departments can openly recruit.
- Opportunistic: Recruiting is allowed if the right candidate comes along.
- No current approval to hire: Recruiting is not approved.

Harborview

Harborview created an international clinic to serve immigrants and refugees with unique needs, including a sizable patient population that had experienced torture. The international clinic includes a large interpretive services program, attendings with global health or anthropology experiences, pharmacy support, and medical assistants (MAs) who speak the predominant languages of these populations. The clinic has a unique pathway that does not include the central access contact center. Patients gain access to the clinic through specialty-care clinics, aftercare plans, and a process that screens refugees when they enter King County.

Stanford Health Care

SHC created several programs to provide immediate access to care, including same-day scheduling clinics (Express Care) and a walk-in clinic that patients can call or message about a new or worsening issue rather than having to go to the emergency department. The Second Opinion Program at SHC (both a stand-alone version and one in partnership with Grand Rounds, a digital-health company) also helps provide access to patients interested in a second opinion. Patients can request a second opinion from SHC specialists knowing that the clinician will respond to their questions within two days and continued communication with the clinician is an option. Data show that of the patients who use the Second Opinion Program, 27% convert to becoming patients at SHC.

SYSTEMWIDE POLICIES AND WORK PROCESSES

Harborview

The first step in the UW's approach to creating a systemwide access strategy was to establish standardized policies across the UW organization within the access governance structure. These standardized policies address cancellations by providers (provider bumps), cancellations by patients, and patient no-shows and are the foundation of the UW access initiative. Stakeholders beyond the access team (e.g., finance, shared services) helped design these standardized, systemwide policies.

Access managers and capacity architects have been key to new, innovative access initiatives at Emory. ... Managers are charged with "owning" access for their divisions much like a financial analyst would "own" the revenue stream.

DATA-DRIVEN PERFORMANCE IMPROVEMENT

Emory

Access managers and capacity architects have been key to new, innovative access initiatives at Emory. Access managers have consistently demonstrated a positive return on investment by expanding access to care and improving performance on no-show rates, schedule optimization, appointment lag (the time between when the appointment was scheduled and when the patient is seen), and patient experience. Managers are charged with "owning" access for their divisions much like a financial analyst would "own" the revenue stream. They review provider data one-on-one with poor performers every month and all providers at least annually. Access managers lift the core culture of patient access and embed it into the divisions at the local level, paving the way for rapid transformative change. Capacity-management architects develop and manage capacity. They are trained to understand the flow and capacity of the clinics and are part of a limited group of individuals who can edit schedules. Although they will not necessarily deny providers' requests for schedule changes, they do provide an impact analysis for recommended or requested changes (e.g., changes in RVU productivity, percentage of new-patient visits, no-show rates).

Leading Practices for Structure and Standard Processes

Centralizing access operations to support scheduling has numerous benefits, and doing it effectively requires prioritizing the patient experience, involving physicians, and creating a supportive structure and standard processes. Many organizations create contact-center operations that include centralized scheduling and nurse-triage capabilities for both primary and specialty care. Other organizations take a more phased approach, adding specialties over time or maintaining some level of decentralization. The type of approach depends on the organization's culture, capacity, and provider readiness for change. Not investing the time and effort to effectively and recurrently engage providers and staff before, during, and after the transition to the centralized system can lead to failure.

CHANGE TACTICS FOR STRUCTURE AND STANDARD PROCESSES

- ☑ Build your case for change to support a centralized call center structure and include physician champions and other key stakeholders in developing your vision and strategy.
- ☑ Implement a formal system for managing schedule changes (e.g., implement a ticket system that includes an approval mechanism). Limit the number of individuals able to change schedules. Initiate ongoing quality-assurance processes to ensure templates function as intended.
- ☑ Implement a pod-scheduling model with a designated scheduling team to address calls from patients requesting specific clinics or practices. Invite providers to visit the call center to meet and develop a relationship with their scheduling team. Create decision trees to help call center staff schedule patients with the correct provider.
- ☑ Review access policies and procedures. Develop a strategy for educating providers about policy changes. Consider creating a "leadership roadshow" for sharing the purpose, scope, objective, and goals of the policies and procedures. When building provider support, focus on the patient experience. Use patient-family advisory councils (PFACs) as a source of patient feedback and engagement.
- ☑ Standardize work processes where you can and customize where you need to. Use established criteria and a decision matrix to recognize when deviating from the standard workflow is appropriate. Involve performance-improvement (PI) staff in identifying process defects as part of improvement activities.
- ☑ Create an infrastructure through dedicated resources and personnel who use data to engage providers, drive culture change, and support sustained improvement efforts. Create scorecards that are visible to all and updated frequently.
- ☑ Empower frontline providers to suggest solutions to improve care. Listen to their recommendations for improvement. Share insights with the PI team.

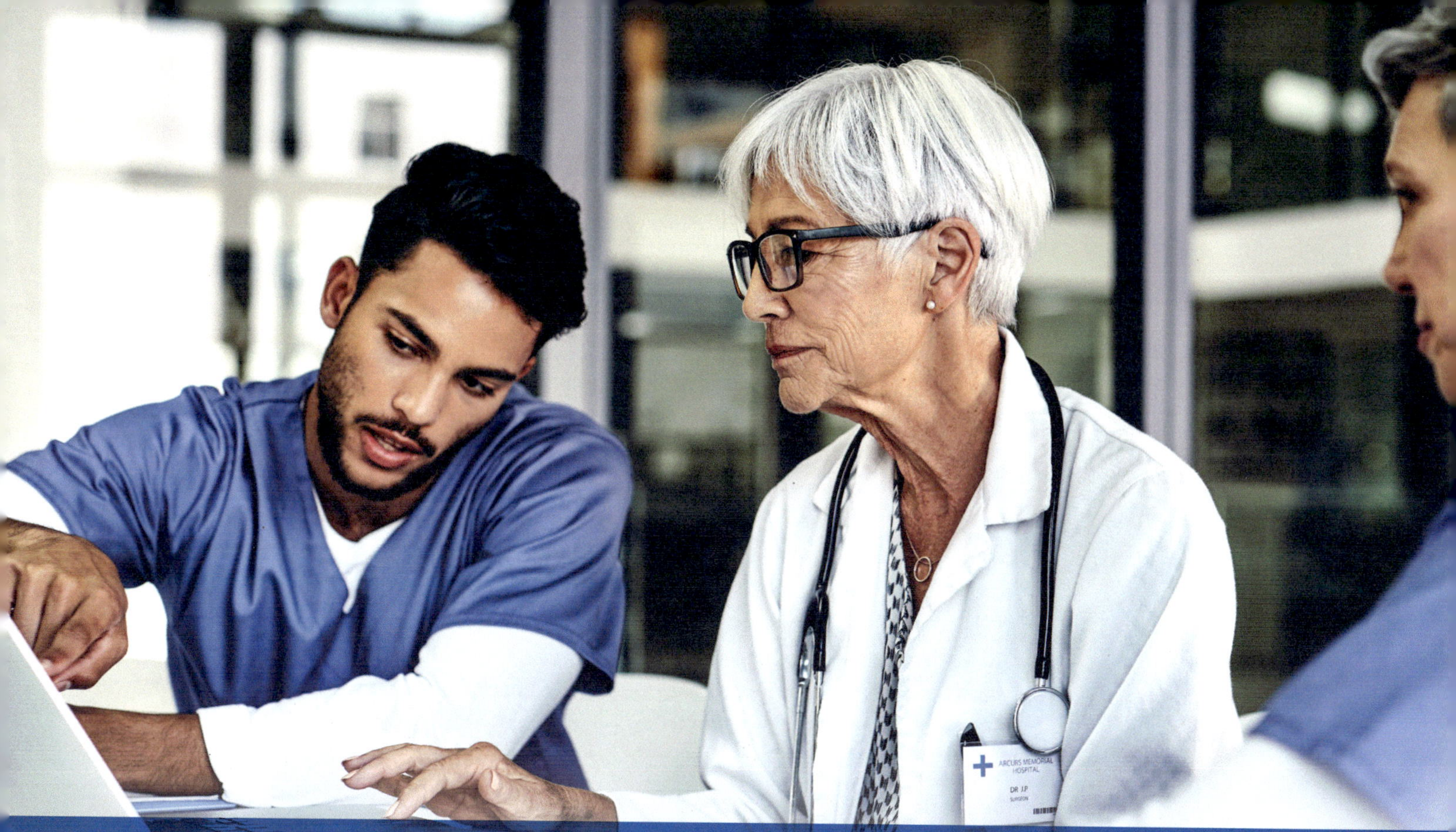

Primary Driver: Actionable Data and Analytics

Simply having data is not enough. What is done with the data sets high performers apart from their competitors. Ensuring data validity, having "relentless attention to detail," as one leader reported, and conducting thoughtful analysis to determine the underlying story lead to the critical steps in improving access.

PRIMARY DRIVER	SECONDARY DRIVERS
Actionable Data and Analytics	**Metric selection and measurement:** Select standard metrics with consistent definitions for measurement and benchmarking.
	Data integrity: Have a process to ensure data are complete, reliable, and timely so providers and leaders can make effective decisions.
	Data reporting and transparency: Support collaborative efforts for continuous improvement through consistent data sharing among leadership, clinics, and providers.

AAMC vizient.

METRIC SELECTION AND MEASUREMENT

Stanford Health Care

SHC created a systemwide, automated patient-access dashboard that reports performance on key metrics related to wait time and missed referrals, utilization, and outputs. The organization uses the metrics to enhance their understanding of demand and supply while also interpreting them through the lens of the patient experience. Top-, clinic-, and other-level performance data are reported for each metric. Benchmark data from the CPSC are included in the access dashboard where appropriate.

Colorado

Active panel management and ensuring every patient is included in a primary care panel have been essential strategies for primary care clinics at Colorado. Various risk categories are used to classify different types of patients seen across clinics and to understand the frequency of visits per patient in each category. Colorado defined six tiers of risk for patients, from low (1.2 visits per year) to high (13.2 visits per year). They use that information to ensure clinic spots are available to meet patient needs. This approach allows Colorado to understand their patient population's needs and to set appropriate clinic panel size.

DATA INTEGRITY

Emory

Emory has invested in a centralized data analytics team that specializes in publishing accurate, actionable, digestible data and data visualizations. The team compiles all the dashboards, from the access dashboard to the telemedicine and other dashboards used daily, as the reliable and central source for performance data. In addition, for the contact center and capacity management, the access team has developed a way to report on real-time access through the access dashboard. Contact-center and capacity-management reports are sent twice daily throughout the entire organization (to staff, physicians, and the dean). These monthly reports provide information on situational awareness, volumes of patients, staffing, and service levels. This transparent, timely data sharing creates the opportunity to adjust workflow changes during the week to address access challenges as they emerge.

The Harborview data are so robust that performance can be examined at a subpopulation level, using race, ethnicity, and language (REAL) data. Being able to study the data and outcomes with an equity lens, inclusive of various social determinants of health, helps Harborview stay true to their mission to care for vulnerable populations.

DATA REPORTING AND TRANSPARENCY

Harborview

Harborview has identified several data metrics to report on in the aggregate and at the clinic and individual provider levels. Harborview leadership believes change requires sharing provider-level data. Clinic administrator-and-provider dyads review the data monthly or more frequently, if needed. The data are shared and posted in the department or clinic, reviewed during leadership rounds, and discussed during the Ambulatory Council monthly meetings. The Harborview data are so robust that performance can be examined at a subpopulation level, using race, ethnicity, and language (REAL) data. Being able to study the data and outcomes with an equity lens, inclusive of various social determinants of health, helps Harborview stay true to their mission to care for vulnerable populations.

NYU

NYU uses data from the CPSC and other sources for their data and analytics platform. The central access team identifies trends, defines performance metrics, sets performance targets by specialty, and measures providers against these targets. Data are shared transparently among practices and used as levers to identify workflow, process, and performance variations and drive change within the organization.

Leading Practices for Actionable Data and Analytics

These organizations use data to drive their work on access. They align their performance metrics with their organizational priorities, set performance targets for each department, and consistently gather data for all departments. They routinely measure and understand performance through visual dashboards (see the appendix for sample metrics). The data infrastructure should enable the grouping and review of individual provider-level data at the clinic, department, and overall organization levels. Provider-level data are essential for engaging individual providers in performance improvement, and department- and clinic-level data are viewed and used by clinical and operational leadership.

CHANGE TACTICS FOR ACTIONABLE DATA AND ANALYTICS

- ☑ Select best-in-class access metrics that align with your organization's strategic priorities. See the appendix for a list of potential metrics to use.
- ☑ Define metrics and benchmarks with the goal of standardizing measurement of performance across the organization. Measure across all specialties with the understanding that targets may differ by specialty. Use data to support change and ongoing improvement efforts.
- ☑ Validate the accuracy of data sources. Scrub data and eliminate noise leading to compromised or corrupt data sets.
- ☑ Create dashboards of performance metrics with targeted goals. Ensure dashboards are available and easily accessible to all key stakeholders (leadership roundtables, departments and clinics, individual providers), ensure individuals are aware of the dashboards, and create incentives for individuals to use them.
- ☑ Conduct routine data-review meetings with executive leadership and clinic managers. Drive provider engagement via transparent and routine data sharing. To identify opportunities for performance improvement, create a formal way for providers to share feedback.

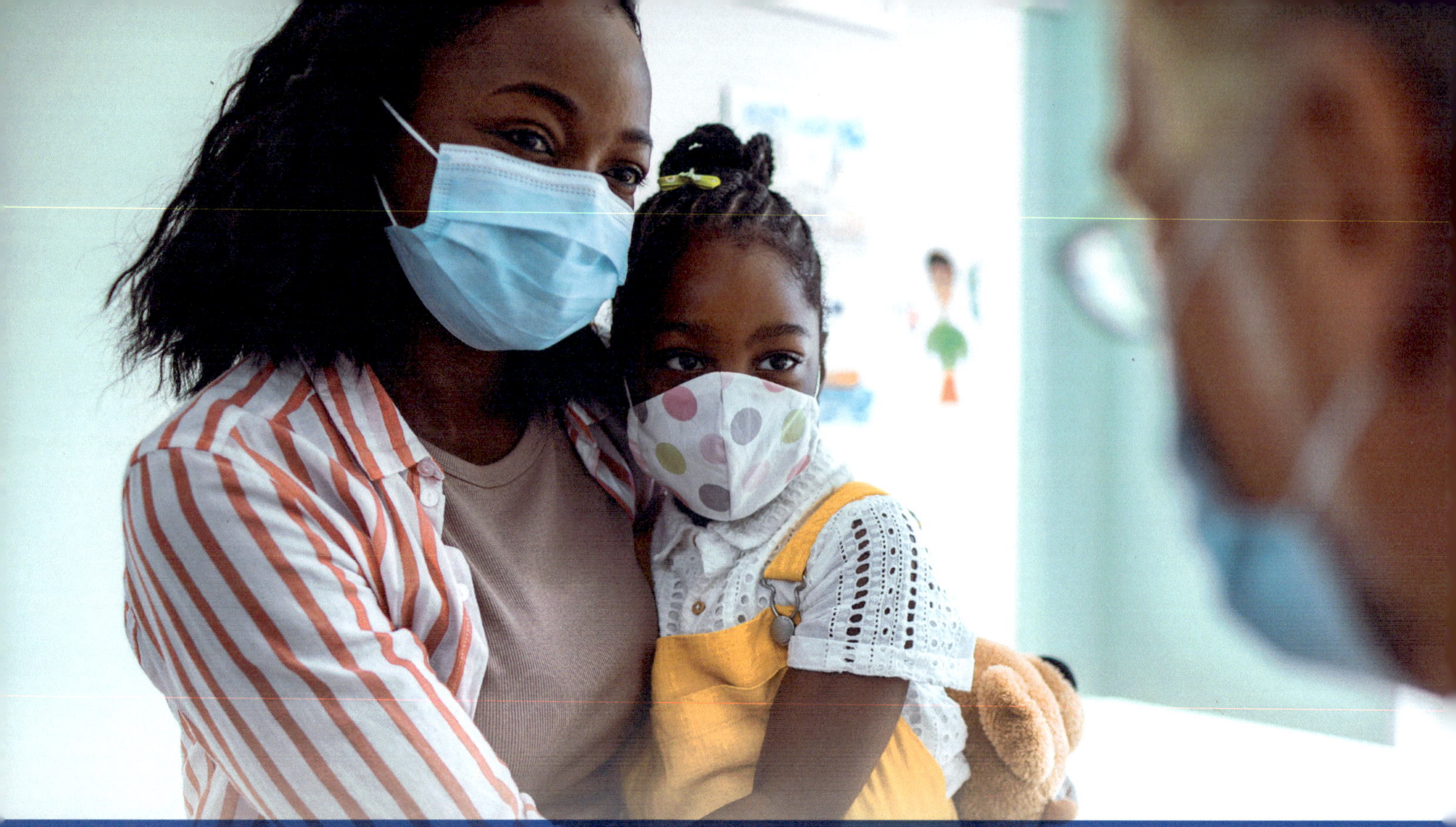

Primary Driver: Optimize Care Delivery

Optimizing care delivery and the care team is crucial to maximizing capacity and improving throughput (the number of patients seen per clinic session) while providing high-quality care. Evaluating the type of care and services provided is essential to understanding the mix of staff needed to deliver care and improve access.

PRIMARY DRIVER	SECONDARY DRIVERS
Optimize Care Delivery	**Team-based care:** Implement a care model that tailors responsibilities and roles to each member of the team to improve productivity and access.
	Population health management: Create ways for staff to understand specific patient subpopulations and target interventions that are distinct to each group to improve the health status of the entire population served by the health system.
	Performance optimization: Understand that care-delivery models are not one-size-fits-all and require evaluation and iteration and consider that customization helps maximize the output of individual providers and others on the care team.
	Equitable, patient-centered care: Prioritize knowing and treating the full patient and providing care that promotes equity and systemic efforts to reduce disparities in health care access, use, and quality.

TEAM-BASED CARE

Stanford Health Care

SHC strives for a goal of a 3,000-to-1 patient-to-doctor ratio in primary care achieved through integrated care teams. In 2014, SCH started a primary care 2.0 design process that included "pods" — partnerships between an MD and an APP with MA support. These pods are supported by a central care team of a clinical pharmacist, nutritionist, behavioral health specialist, and physical therapist. Within UHA, efforts to optimize team-based care have focused on:

- Pre-visit preparation and abstraction (gathering data from lab and imaging reports).
- Daily meetings with the provider and the MA.
- Patient workflows in clinic, including the rooming process.
- MA-to-provider handoff.
- Management of providers' work in the EMR and offline beyond the visit (in-basket and offline-work management).
- MA as flow manager.

SHC has also worked to find the most effective use of scribes. Many organizations struggle with scribe turnover. SHC faculty practice clinics that emphasize teaching have found the most effective model to use for scribes is a fellowship for future medical school applicants; community clinics that tend to have higher volumes of patients use employed scribes. Once clinics reach a volume and productivity threshold, they strategize about the appropriate model for their scribes and implement a service-level agreement to meet their financial and productivity goals. The effective use of scribes has freed up other team members, including RNs.

Colorado

Colorado found that implementing team-based care in primary care and select specialty practices allowed for more innovation and higher productivity across the care team. They use a ratio of 5:2 MAs to physicians. The MAs work side-by-side with the physicians and serve as scribes. An MA institute was developed to educate staff about this elevated scope of work, including roles and responsibilities, and serves as a retention strategy. The MAs feel their role is more important and meaningful in this new structure, and staff turnover rates have decreased. Within primary care, this model has allowed the number of new patients per month to double and the panel size to increase without extending the time for a new appointment. Colorado's team-based approach also includes care managers, social workers, and dieticians in nearly all primary care clinics. APPs are used in most specialties, including pulmonology and gastroenterology. Initially, pulmonologists and APPs shared a panel of patients. As trust developed, APPs transitioned to having their own panel of patients to manage. In gastroenterology, APPs see clinic patients, while physicians spend time in the lab and on research.

POPULATION HEALTH MANAGEMENT

Emory

At the Emory Diabetes Center, a team dedicated to treating patients with diabetes identifies patients whose diabetes is poorly controlled and initiates outreach through the patients' providers. Patients are invited to participate in a program designed to optimize patient care. For about 12 months, they have separate visits with a diabetes nurse practitioner (NP), who focuses on the diabetes part of their care, and a PCP, who coordinates other aspects of their care. Patients receive more frequent and ongoing care and coaching than they would with their regular provider and more opportunities for updates to their treatment plan between visits with the PCP. The ongoing connection with a disease-focused management team provides better continuity of care and prepares patients for physician visits.

Colorado

CU Medicine, the faculty practice plan that supports the medical school providers, sponsors the Office of Value-Based Performance (OVBP), the home for the work that supports population health and value-based programs. OVBP uses data to gain insights into procedures, immunizations, and diagnoses to better understand patient care needs. Housed within OVBP, the Ambulatory Health Promotion program extends outreach to patients for evidence-based preventive services (e.g., breast and colon cancer screening) and treatment for chronic conditions such as diabetes and depression. Outreach coordinators improve patient access to care by contacting patients and working to close any care gaps by creating multiple access points for patient care. The coordinators ensure patients with acute needs who need to be seen by a provider are seen in an appropriate care setting (e.g., in the emergency department or with their PCP). Patients with chronic yet stable conditions are supported and managed through ongoing outreach efforts from the outreach coordinator between visits.

PERFORMANCE OPTIMIZATION

NYU

NYU created a practice liaison position in its large multispecialty locations that reports to the access team and, indirectly, to the practice managers. The liaison works closely with management of the practice and frontline staff to pilot new initiatives and policy changes, create corresponding content, develop the communication plan, and coordinate execution and delivery to ensure a successful implementation. This role has been linked to an improvement in access and patient-satisfaction metrics.

Colorado

At Colorado, primary care leadership established the role of practice-transformation champions, individuals in each clinic who focus on teamwork and serve as liaisons among medical directors, practice managers, and MAs across primary care. This role is different from the typical Performance Improvement and Lean method of support (PI/Lean) because it focuses on helping implement changes and guiding the transformation process through team building, re-evaluation, and flexibility.

Colorado has also attempted to expand primary care practice transformation with MA staffing to specialty practices such as gastroenterology. Through this, they learned that one way to maintain sustainability is knowing when to abandon an unworkable approach. The GI physicians spend most of their time doing procedures in the GI lab and, typically, have only one-half clinic session per week. The GI providers quickly realized standardizing the workflow with an increased number of MAs was difficult. They did not maintain the 5:2 MA:physician staffing model standardized as part of the practice transformation; instead, they reassigned the additional support from MAs to focus on contacting patients ahead of time to reduce lab no-shows. While Colorado had success implementing the practice-transformation model in many areas, in others, they followed the adage, "standardize what you can; customize what you have to."

EQUITABLE, PATIENT-CENTERED CARE

Harborview

Harborview created several clinics for patients from populations that may have challenges accessing care in typical clinic settings, such as centers for patients with high viral loads of HIV, a clinic for sex workers, and a safe, healthy, empowerment of women (SHE) clinic. Harborview established strong community partnerships to deliver patient-centered care, including:

- Partnering with supportive housing to embed nurses who can provide care to unhoused people at the right time in the right setting and more cost-effectively than emergency departments.
- Coordinating with and offering telehealth services to jails, focusing on people previously diagnosed as HIV-positive, and developing ongoing care-management programs.
- Adding two clinical social workers in primary care who focus on behavioral health and food, housing, and transportation, respectively, and coordinate care with community partners.

At Emory, physicians and administrators make it a priority to tell stories about their patients to bring providers and staff along on the access journey and drive change within the organization.

Emory

Emory emphasizes patient-centered care through their commitment to grant patients' requests to be seen today, tomorrow, or within one week. When making strategic decisions, Emory seeks the input of patient-family advisory councils. To support a patient-centered approach, Emory asks each division to define and operationally support what "expedited access" can be for that division. For example, some divisions define this as clinical acuity (the level of care and support needed), while others rely more on provider and patient expectations. After the division defines patient eligibility for "expedited access," the access and operations teams support that access through schedule design and infrastructure that includes marketing specific phone numbers to the public to increase the number of calls to the call center. Physicians and administrators make it a priority to tell stories about their patients to bring providers and staff along on the access journey and drive change within the organization.

Leading Practices for Optimized Care Delivery

Many organizations consistently emphasize using team-based-care models in primary and specialty care. What set the five organizations selected for this report apart was how they implemented these models: They used a novel approach that includes designating team members to support effective clinical redesign and related efforts to optimize access and throughput. These individuals have various titles — capacity-management architect, practice liaison, practice-transformation champion — but they all focus on engaging with providers in day-to-day work. They work with providers to implement performance-improvement interventions that address access challenges.

CHANGE TACTICS FOR OPTIMIZED CARE DELIVERY

- ☑ Clearly delineate roles in clinics, with defined roles and responsibilities of each clinical provider type. Ensure team members are working at the top of their license.
- ☑ Map workflows to identify team members' roles. Implement standard workflows to assist the interdisciplinary team with pre-visit-planning, visit, and after-visit tasks.
- ☑ Prioritize considering access to care with a health-equity lens. Consider the specific needs of different segments of your patient population. Screen for social determinants of health and mobilize team members to deliver care within the appropriate care setting.
- ☑ When designing an individual care plan and providing care, use a patient-centered approach that includes the patient's preferences, needs, and values.
- ☑ Use data from multiple sources to support population health efforts. Analyze the data to find insights into procedures, immunizations, and diagnoses that can inform how care is delivered and address patient needs across a population.
- ☑ Build and strengthen relationships with community-based organizations, governmental entities, and physician affiliations to promote access in the community setting. Use the resources and expertise of the AMC to develop provider-to-provider education programs for sharing leading practices and improving care delivery.
- ☑ Understand the limits of scaling a fixed model (e.g., the 5:2 MA:physician team-based-care model). Evaluate your approach so you can modify it, if necessary, in local and specialty-specific contexts.
- ☑ For successful change management, establish a role for individuals who are implementing workflow changes, guiding change, building teams, evaluating results, and helping clinics improve adaptability.

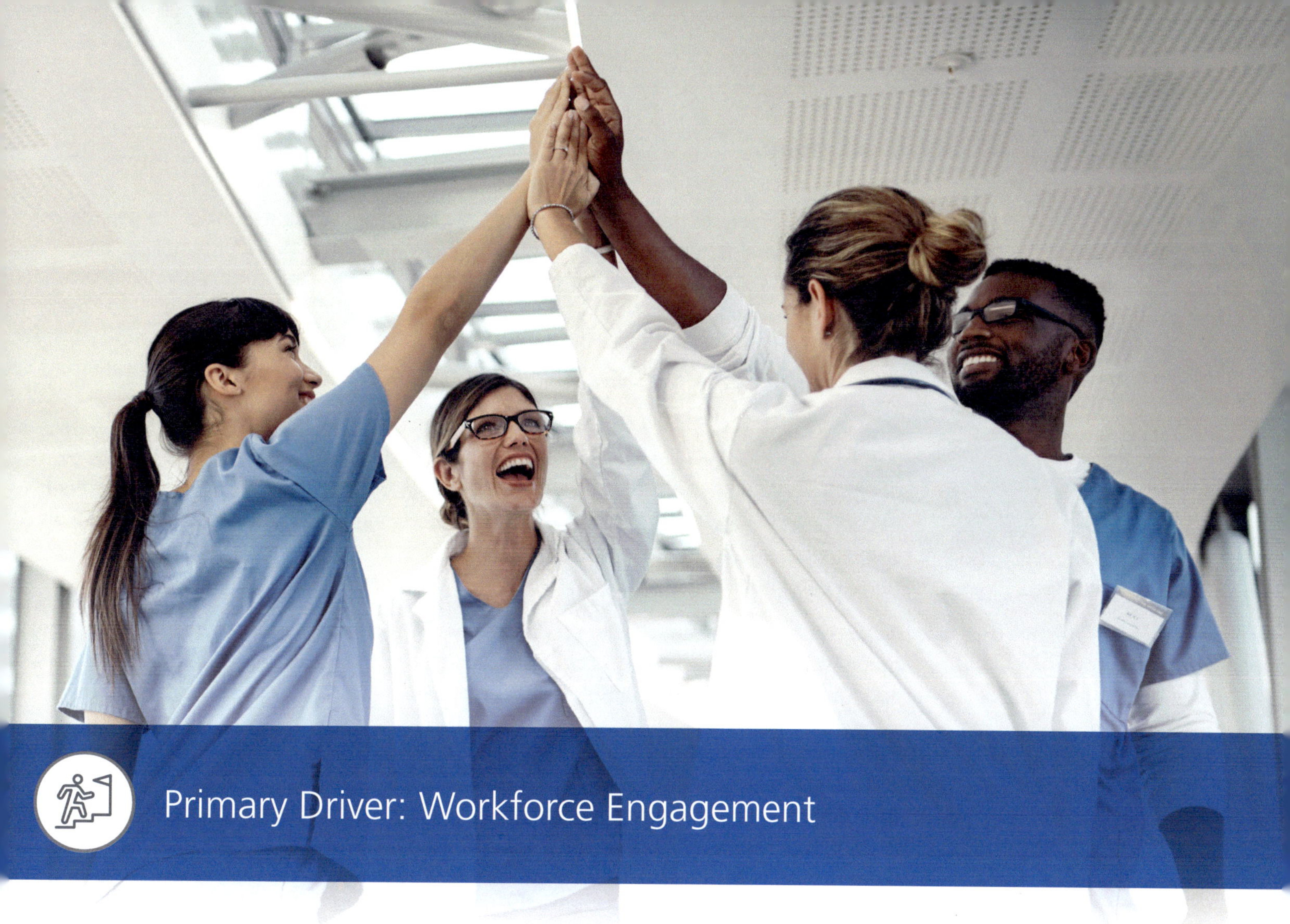

Primary Driver: Workforce Engagement

Increasing workforce engagement involves reducing turnover, building skills, fostering community, and aligning with the access goals of the organization. Engagement begins with onboarding and continues with sharing data, building accountability, and ensuring high levels of competency. Success is rewarded, and incentive structures motivate the workforce to exceed expectations aligned with the shared mission, vision, and values set by the leadership team.

PRIMARY DRIVER	SECONDARY DRIVERS
Workforce Engagement	**Onboarding:** Uses an organizational approach with role-specific programs that help the care team gain the knowledge, skills, and cultural behaviors necessary to be effective.
	Education and training: Schedules longitudinal forums at regular intervals to provide teaching, learning, and best-practice sharing for staff and providers.
	Incentives, recognition, and rewards: Develops official programs to recognize team members and clinics for improving, achieving organizational goals, and demonstrating the organization's cultural behaviors and values.

AAMC vizient.

ONBOARDING

Emory

Historically at Emory, as new providers joined the group, they would meet with the department secretary to develop their schedule. This led to wide variation in provider templates and scheduling. In 2009, standardization efforts began, with the access administrative team proactively meeting with each individual provider as part of the onboarding process. The scope of each provider's practice, including unique aspects and guardrails (e.g., productivity targets such as RVUs) are discussed to create the ideal scheduling template for meeting the provider's needs. The view at Emory is that physicians "own" access. They have the flexibility to build their ideal schedule if it meets their department's access goals. However, if the "ideal" day does not materialize, provider templates become more flexible close to the date of clinic; provider blocks and preferences are removed, allowing any appointment to book at any time. The administrative team supports the access journey through protocols and templates. This process balances provider preference and optimizing access, and it has been a good tradeoff for the Emory team.

Beyond provider onboarding, the access mentorship program matches people early in their career with a mentor from the access team. Mentors help mentees build confidence, network, and learn specific skills to realize their full potential.

Stanford Health Care

The Center for Advanced Practice at SHC has seen notable variation in the roles and use of APPs across faculty and UHA practices. To address this variation, SHC created the APP SHINE program, which heightens the integration and engagement of APPs. Clinical department chairs help determine whether an APP is ready to practice independently. The goal of the program is to increase the understanding of how APPs are being used and to standardize their use. SHC has found that within primary care, developing a sense of team and wellness is essential to effectively engaging APPs. Effective MD-APP partnerships have three attributes:

- **Effective communication through in-person discussion, by secure messaging, or over the phone, with dedicated time for it.**
- **Mutual respect, which takes time to develop and reduces redundancy in checking documentation and diagnostic testing.**
- **Shared philosophy of care. MD-APP dyads must have complementary practice styles and clinical alignment.**

Colorado

Colorado has invested time and resources in the onboarding and development of APPs. The hospital launched the Office of Advanced Practice (OAP) five years ago, which was jointly funded through the medical school and UCHealth. Working with the department vice-chairs of clinical affairs, the OAP created a learning module to educate physicians about the APP scope of practice and examples of how APPs are used. After that, each specialty developed a "roles and responsibilities" document to standardize expectations for team members, including attendings, fellows, residents, students, and APPs. The OAP provides a professional development coordinator, who develops an onboarding plan for each new provider with follow-ups at one, three, six, and nine months. This process has created a professional home for the APPs and fostered a culture of team-based care. A departmental lead APP role was created within this structure to give the APPs a voice and representation within the individual departments. The University Hospital Board allows APPs to be nominated for elected positions, and two APPs have served on the board to date.

EDUCATION AND TRAINING

Harborview

Harborview has leveraged Project ECHO (Extension for Community Healthcare Outcomes, a national program) to support their access strategy by focusing on educating and training PCPs in the WWAMI region (Washington, Wyoming, Alaska, Montana, and Idaho). The project increases the capacity for community providers to care for underserved populations in the patient's own community. Harborview faculty and regional providers have weekly conference calls, during which academic physicians share their expertise with regional community providers to help patients avoid unnecessary travel to Harborview.

NYU

NYU has created weekly educational forums to highlight and reinforce the strategic priorities of the organization. Topics include front-end operations, access optimization, and best practices in access and operations. These sessions, hosted virtually, in classrooms, or both, include training in customer service skills, template management, managed care, how to make referrals, how to handle provider cancellations, and other requested subjects. In addition to the weekly educational sessions, NYU has established patient-experience, patient-access, and clinical workgroups as channels for providing education and training. The workgroups create a supportive environment in which participants from different practices and different roles can discuss successes and challenges. The workgroups focus on sharing best practices, trying new methods, and scaling up methods across the organization.

INCENTIVES, RECOGNITION, AND REWARDS

Emory

As part of optimizing access for providers, Emory created an access-focused, division-level incentive, the Shared Operational Unit Performance (SOUP). The division chooses an access-focused metric (e.g., rate of provider cancellation) and sets specific performance targets. When those targets are met, the division receives an incentive to use for projects (not salaries). SOUP shows leadership commitment to improving access. Emory also uses access metrics in its senior management incentive program (SMIP), with at least 15% of every senior leader's incentive payout based on the access metric performance in their division. Aligning administrative and clinical incentive programs allows Emory to focus on and reach ambitious access goals.

Emory's Recognizing Exceptional Support of Patient Experience in Challenging Times (RESPECT) program incentivizes team members through positive reinforcement and gamification to have perfect attendance on Mondays and Tuesdays (the highest call-volume days). Team members who meet the eligibility criteria receive "E-Recognize" points that allow them to purchase items from an online catalog. Emory has also created a quarterly "shark tank" innovation that allows team members (supervisor level and below) to draft project pitches to improve the experience of staff or patients. Team members pitch their idea to the "sharks" (leadership team members), who fund the winning idea with both time and dollars.

NYU

NYU uses key metrics — such as number of new patients in 10 days, number of no-shows, and percentage of people enrolling in the patient portal, MyChart — to recognize top-performing faculty practices and individuals. At the regional level, high performers are honored at rewards and recognition programs such as a winner's lunch, and trophies are given to high and most-improved performers. This creates an environment of healthy competition and honors and reinforces a commitment to workgroup excellence.

Leading Practices for Workforce Engagement

While organizational culture around improving access to care is set and reinforced by engaged leaders, improving access also requires that individual providers and staff throughout the organization understand and extend the organization's commitment to it. The selected organizations have achieved this understanding and extension of commitment to access through formalized workforce engagement during onboarding, ongoing training efforts, and rewards and recognition programs tied to achieving access goals.

CHANGE TACTICS FOR WORKFORCE ENGAGEMENT

- ☑ Create formalized onboarding programs uniquely designed for each provider type, including frontline staff; clinical providers such as MAs, nurses, and APPs; and physicians. Assess competence after training to identify gaps.
- ☑ Deploy an access team to meet with physicians and other clinical providers to discuss scope and purpose of practice, clinic expectations, and cultural norms.
- ☑ Provide opportunities for peer-to-peer learning, networking, mentoring, and best-practice sharing. Design role-specific educational opportunities and conduct weekly trainings for contact-center and clinic staff. Develop modules for clinical leadership training on the roles, responsibilities, and use of APPs.
- ☑ Incentivize high performance on access-driven metrics in addition to volume-driven metrics. Allocate funds back to departments that meet their performance goals. Develop APP incentives built around independent visits and panel management. Align incentives and performance appraisals to drive the access strategy and overall performance.
- ☑ Celebrate performance milestones on key metrics by creating monthly clinic awards. Recognize clinic staff who are leading performers and most improved. Create reward and recognition programs that reinforce the values and goals of your organization.
- ☑ Host leadership roundtables with staff, such as breakfast or lunch meetings, to encourage discussions about successes, challenges, and opportunities at work. Reinforce the access culture among staff by encouraging direct interaction with executive leadership.

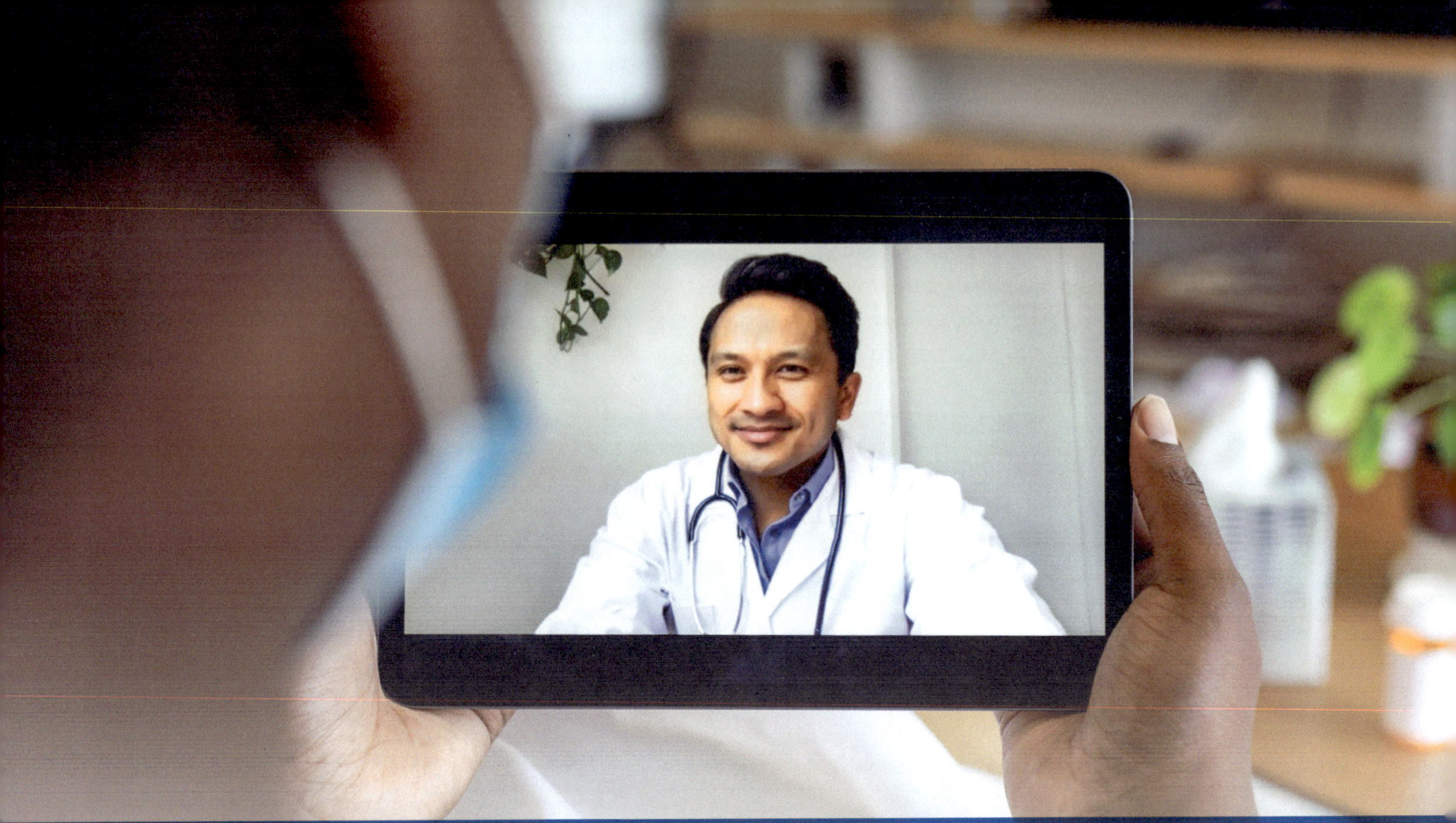

Primary Driver: Leverage Technology

Leveraging technology to meet patients' demands around convenience, quality, and timeliness of access to care can powerfully improve access and patients' experience. Navigating the digital world has become second nature to most patients, and they now expect health care organizations to use technology to support communication, care coordination, and care delivery. Meeting patients where they are is an important access strategy, which, in the case of technology, requires ingenuity and the seamless application of technological advances.

PRIMARY DRIVER	SECONDARY DRIVERS
Leverage Technology	**EMR optimization:** Customize and use the EMR strategically to create workflows to address care-delivery needs.
	Virtual health capabilities: Optimize telehealth and technology to deliver care at a distance across a range of settings.
	Digital front door: Create a single, simple way for patients to gain access to the health care organization.
	Artificial intelligence and predictive analytics: Use data mining to help with referral management and care delivery.

AAMC vizient.

EMR OPTIMIZATION

NYU

NYU has worked over the years to optimize the functionality of the EMR for patients and providers and to streamline processes that facilitate improved access to care. For example, they created check-in kiosks that build on the EMR to improve the check-in experience. These changes have freed up front-desk staff to improve the patient experience by focusing on more-complex tasks and high-touch activities. Other improvements NYU has implemented include an automated waitlist option that enables patients to move up appointments and a recall feature that reminds them to schedule an appointment. Overall, NYU approaches the EMR by attempting to understand and maximize its abilities to align with operations functions, which leads to improvements in operational effectiveness.

Stanford Health Center

SHC has fully embraced the tools and capabilities offered within the EMR. The organization implemented an automated waitlist system that offers appointments to patients at midnight based on open slots that day. They typically have 25 waitlist visits per day and 6,300 per year. SHC's patient portal, MyHealth, has played a key role in actively engaging patients. MyHealth is built on top of the EMR's standard patient portal, and almost 90% of primary care patients are enrolled in the portal. The key to this level of enrollment has been changing the expectation from "please use" to "this is how providers and the care team communicate with patients." This has been an important step for Stanford in expanding their digital offerings.

SHC's patient portal, MyHealth, has played a key role in actively engaging patients. MyHealth is built on top of the EMR's standard patient portal, and almost 90% of primary care patients are enrolled in the portal. The key to this level of enrollment has been changing the expectation from "please use" to "this is how providers and the care team communicate with patients."

Colorado

Using the EMR platform to its full capability has been central to Colorado's access initiatives. They have leveraged all the tools available in the EMR, from incorporating the EMR's population health management module to creating eConsults through the AAMC's Project CORE (Coordinating Optimal Referral Experiences), to using all the features of the patient portal and self-scheduling. They included decision trees in the EMR to support team-based scheduling and to determine whether a visit should be virtual or in person. To enhance physician confidence in the system, Colorado developed a feedback mechanism that captures scheduling errors, and the contact center reviews and responds to feedback within 24 hours. UCH has developed teams that work directly with clinics to optimize EMR workflows and with providers to improve comfort with EMR tools that can streamline clinical care and documentation.

VIRTUAL HEALTH CAPABILITIES

Harborview

Harborview has created five main categories of telehealth. Synchronous video and chat have made possible psychiatric visits in counties that do not have psychiatric providers and for the county jail. As participants in Project CORE, eConsults were established in 2016 to provide patients with improved access to specialty care and support primary care with timely input and expertise from specialists. Harborview also focused on mobile health, remote patient monitoring, and participating in Project ECHO to help support and train community providers.

Stanford Health Care

SHC uses four considerations when determining when and where to go digital: "personalize access, connect networks, transform value, and empower care teams." They are growing their many virtual care programs, including for pre- and post-procedure follow-up, longitudinal care visits, emergency department triage, and eConsults through Project CORE.

Colorado

Colorado has been expanding virtual health visits across primary care. During the scheduling process, they attempt to identify opportunities for virtual health visits. For example, a patient arrives at the clinic and an MA assesses the patient's technical capabilities and readiness for a potential virtual visit. The physician then determines whether a tele-encounter is clinically appropriate. As part of the check-out procedure, the patient receives two appointments with the physician, one for a video visit and the other for a subsequent in-person visit.

DIGITAL FRONT DOOR

NYU

NYU has invested in the development and marketing of its patient digital-access tools, including the patient portal and the internet, which new and existing patients can use 24/7 to schedule appointments. The multifaceted marketing campaign includes using commercials, billboards, and waiting room advertisements to engage patients with NYU's applications and online platform.

Stanford Health Care

SHC is developing a fully digital "front door" with personalized access. They have found that building on the EMR application is essential to making it more user-friendly and customized to SHC. They hope to create an "air traffic control system" that can be paired with the digital front door to ensure patients are seeing the right provider. The patient experience is at the forefront of any digital modification or expansion, with user interface development conducted through a partnership between technical and nontechnical teams that incorporate feedback from patients and families into the design of the system.

ARTIFICIAL INTELLIGENCE AND PREDICTIVE ANALYTICS

Emory

Emory has implemented software to help patients find an ideal provider. Patients can search using specialty- and condition-specific terms to be matched with the ideal provider. Emory is also looking into AI-supported chatbots and online scheduling tools.

NYU

NYU has added the ability for patients to use search terms to find the right providers when they schedule appointments online. A priority in this process has been narrowing the clinical focus of providers to better match patients with their ideal provider. The access team partners with clinical leadership to lead this process by using their operational knowledge in conjunction with their review of specialty- and provider-level billing codes. The access team continuously refines and optimizes what is available to patients online and how best to direct patients to the right provider.

Leading Practices for Leveraging Technology

A common theme across these systems is reliance on a single, standardized EMR platform across all practices to link scheduling, patient data, and patient portals. The EMR is a vehicle for standardizing and supporting a care infrastructure that allows access to be at the forefront. A standardized EMR allows scheduling to be centralized across clinics while also enabling patients to schedule appointments. It also facilitates communication and coordination between care teams and serves as the platform on which future virtual health capabilities can be expanded, especially those that use big data to improve processes that promote better access and customized services.

CHANGE TACTICS FOR LEVERAGING TECHNOLOGY

- ☑ Standardize the EMR platform across all practices and capitalize on EMR capabilities to support access efforts, including patient self-service tools.
- ☑ Identify services for which virtual health visits are appropriate and use telehealth to manage capacity and throughput in clinic.
- ☑ Explore and create telehealth models in the synchronous, asynchronous, provider-patient, and provider-provider settings.
- ☑ Develop web- or app-based tools to help patients find providers. Create targeted outreach campaigns to promote awareness and use of the patient portal.
- ☑ Consider using remote-monitoring tools and technology to support the management of chronic disease care. Create appropriate clinic workflows to review data and proactively manage patients.
- ☑ Modernize IT capabilities to review multiple data sources to identify gaps in care, which supports clinical decision-making.

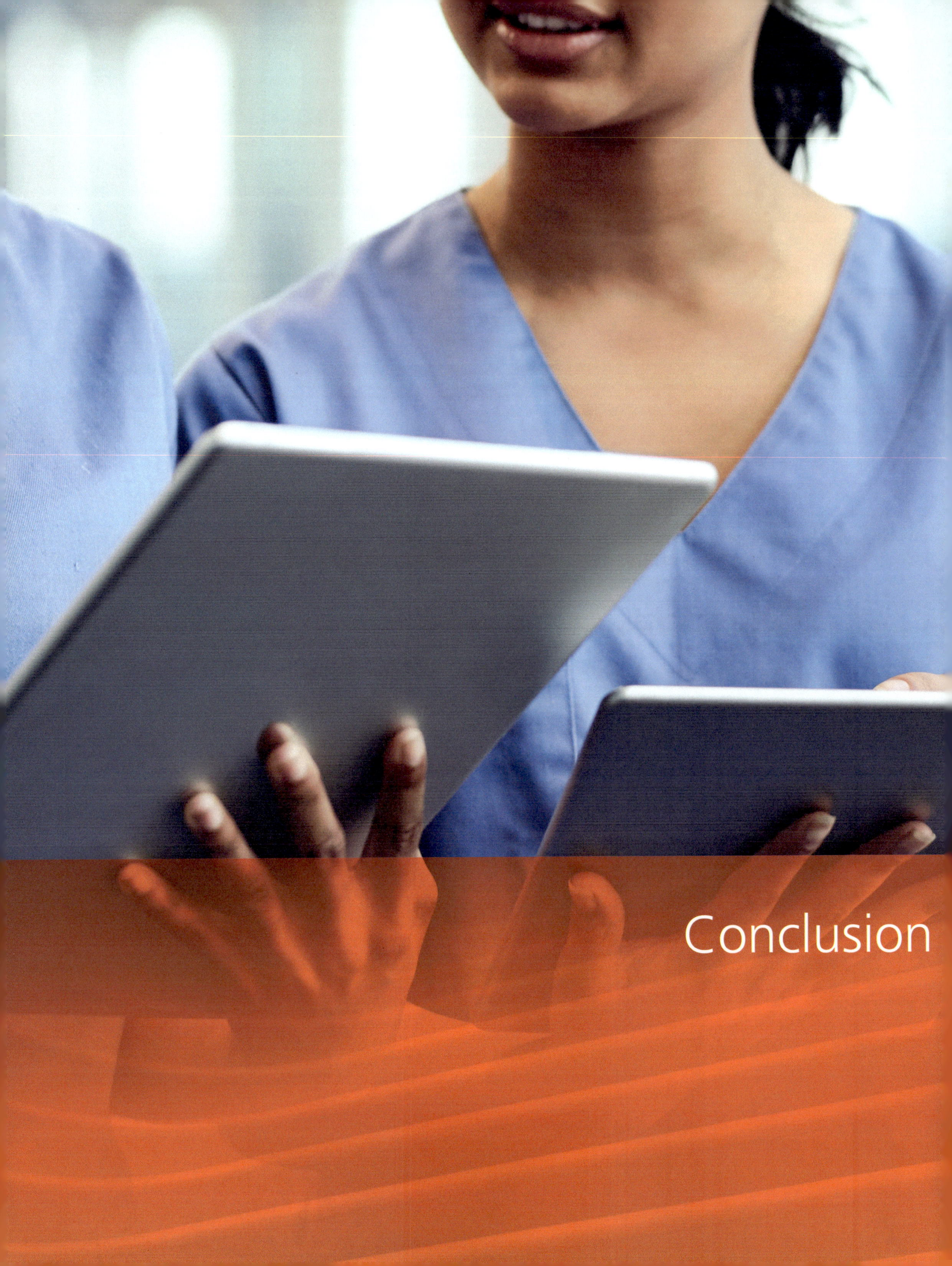

Conclusion

A commitment to improving access to care within the system is a central component of most health care organizations' strategies. Providing quality care is critical but insufficient without adequate access to care. This document provides examples of leading strategies exemplar organizations use to improve patient access. These organizations' high ranking in the Access domain in the Vizient Ambulatory Quality and Accountability Scorecard indicates their leadership's commitment to improving patient access.

As demonstrated in this report, leadership is foundational to the access journey. A common theme across all the highlighted organizations is the existence of a dedicated access leader who is accountable to the organization's access strategy and goals. The organizations also created a culture that prioritizes a patient-centered approach to access to care. These efforts are supported by organization-wide standard processes that optimize care delivery and lead to a cohesive and engaged workforce.

Technology has changed the way patients interact with and seek health care services, particularly during the COVID-19 pandemic. While this technology does not replace in-person contact, it is an increasingly central component of care coordination, delivery, and improved access. Critical components of the access framework are establishing key indicators for measuring access performance and identifying opportunities for improving access. These components should be aligned with incentives to drive continuous performance-improvement efforts. Finally, COVID-19 has brought into sharp focus the extent to which social disparities and inequities in health and health care access persist. Now more than ever, equitable access to health care should be at the forefront of every health care conversation. You can adapt the access framework, associated change tactics, and examples presented in this report to help your organization improve patient access.

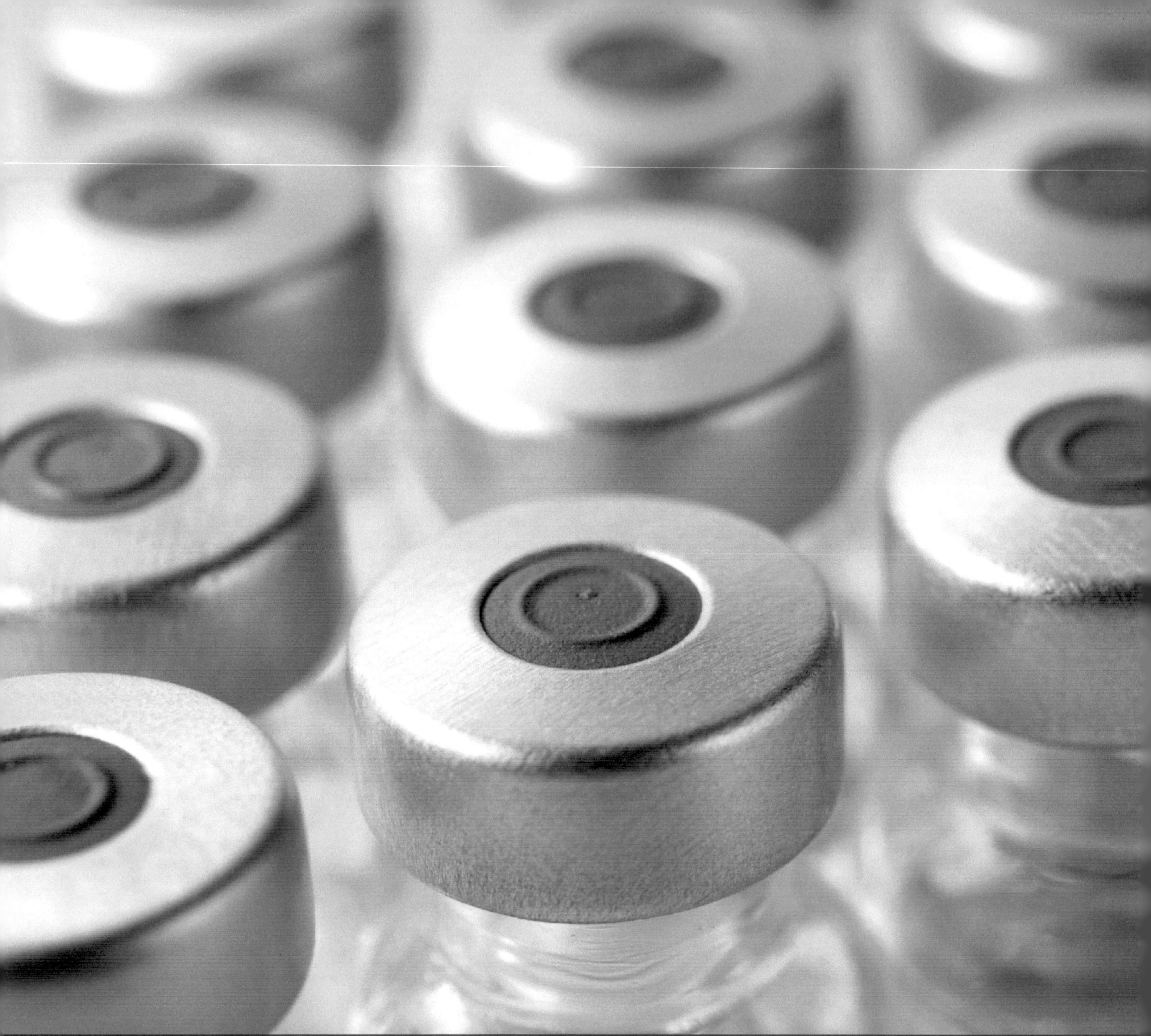

COVID-19 Addendum

The work that led to this report began in May 2019, and the site visits were completed in December 2019. Consequently, this document is focused on the access challenges and initiatives to improve access in a pre-COVID-19 world. The COVID-19 pandemic significantly altered the health care landscape. Health care systems throughout the country have been forced to adapt to meet patients' shifting needs and demands. The following are key areas where COVID-19 has caused a shift in access priorities and interventions:

- Evaluation of overarching ambulatory access strategy.
- Acceleration of virtual care delivery.
- New manifestations of health inequities for vulnerable populations.
- Redesigned patient workflows and processes (that is, patients' experience in the clinic).
- New and changing access points.
- Fluctuating patient demand.
- Workforce engagement and resilience.

Despite the changed health care landscape, the access framework and drivers outlined in this document remain relevant and provide actionable tactics for improving access before, during, and after a pandemic. Recognizing the impact this pandemic has had on academic health systems, the AAMC and Vizient will continue to explore academic health system challenges and the resulting innovations and to share lessons learned and leading practices in future work.

NOTES

1. Institute of Medicine. *Access to Health Care in America.* Washington, DC: National Academies Press; 1993. Available at Google Scholar. Accessed Oct. 6, 2020.

2. Vespa J, Medina L, Armstrong DM. Demographic Turning Points for the United States: Population Projections for 2020 to 2060 Population Estimates and Projections Current Population Reports. February 2020. https://www.census.gov/content/dam/Census/library/publications/2020/demo/p25-1144.pdf. Accessed Oct. 6, 2020

3. IHS Markit Ltd. *The Complexities of Physician Supply and Demand: Projections From 2018 to 2033.* Washington, DC: AAMC; 2020. https://www.aamc.org/system/files/2020-06/stratcomm-aamc-physician-workforce-projections-june-2020.pdf. Accessed Oct. 6, 2020.

4. Median wait time in days in 2019 for these 17 specialties, as measured by the Vizient Ambulatory and Quality and Accountability Scorecard, is from the Clinical Practice Solutions Center, clinicalpracticesolutionscenter.org, accessed Nov. 10, 2020: Cardiology; Dermatology; Ears, Nose, and Throat; Endocrinology; Gastroenterology and Hepatology; Hematology and Oncology; Infectious Disease; Nephrology; Neurology; Obstetrics and Gynecology; Ophthalmology; Orthopaedics; Primary Care; Pulmonology; Rheumatology; Surgery; and Urology.

5. National Public Radio, Robert Wood Johnson Foundation, Harvard T.H. Chan School of Public Health. Patients' Perspectives on Health Care in the United States: A Look at Seven States and the Nation. https://www.npr.org/assets/img/2016/02/26/PatientPerspectives.pdf. Accessed Oct. 6, 2020.

6. AAMC, Vizient. *Learning and Leading in Access to Care: An Overview of Member Collaboratives From the AAMC and Vizient.* Washington, DC: AAMC and Vizient; 2019. https://store.aamc.org/learning-and-leading-in-access-to-care-an-overview-of-member-collaboratives-from-the-aamc-and-vizient.html.

7. The 17 specialties measured in the Vizient Ambulatory and Quality and Accountability Scorecard: Cardiology; Dermatology; Ears, Nose, and Throat; Endocrinology; Gastroenterology and Hepatology; Hematology and Oncology; Infectious Disease; Nephrology; Neurology; Obstetrics and Gynecology; Ophthalmology; Orthopaedics; Primary Care; Pulmonology; Rheumatology; Surgery; and Urology.

APPENDIX. DASHBOARD MEASURES TO TRACK

The table below lists typical measures the organizations highlighted in this document use for each clinic functional area. Incorporating these into a scorecard or dashboard, with agreed-upon targets, and sharing them regularly, will provide the necessary framework for successful efforts to improve patient access.

Table A.1. Dashboard Measures to Track, by Functional Area

FUNCTIONAL AREA	MEASURE
Access metrics	Appointment canceled by provider or clinic (bumped) within 30 days of appointment date (% of total appointments)
	Average 2nd-, 3rd-, and 5th-next-available appointment for new patients
	Completed scheduled visits (%)
	Fill rate (%)
	Median encounters per provider per hour
	New patients seen within 10 days of scheduling appointment (%)
	New-patient median lag (days)
	New-patient scheduling lag (days)
	New-patient visits (% of total visits)
	No-show appointments for same- or previous-day cancellations preceding appointment (%)
	No-show rate (%)
	Overbook rate (%)
	Reschedule rate (%)
	Same-day cancellation rate (%)
	Total visits
	Unfilled same-day cancellations (%)
Phone management	Abandonment rate (%)
	Appointments, reschedules, and cancellations
	Appointments scheduled via centralized contact center (%)
	Average handle time (RN) (minutes)
	Average speed to answer (RN) (minutes)
	Call hold > 60 seconds
	Call-to-visit ratios
	Phone call answer rate (%)
	Prescription-refill rate (%)
	Referrals
	Service-level calls to RNs answered within 30 minutes
	Total handled call volume
	Total incoming call volume
	Transfers

(continued)

Table A.1. Dashboard Measures to Track, by Functional Area *(continued)*

FUNCTIONAL AREA	MEASURE
Quality outcomes	Blood pressure control in hypertensive patients Diabetes: reduce HbA1c poor control
Referral management	Active referrals Average days to first patient contact Average days in pending clinical review Average days to scheduled appointment Leakage (%) Median new-patient-visit-referral creation to appointment (days) Referral age in calendar days Referral completion rate (% of referrals that result in a visit)
Satisfaction	Clinic's access-to-care Clinician and Group Consumer Assessment of Healthcare Providers and Systems (CG-CAHPS) Employee retention rate (%)

Made in United States
Cleveland, OH
05 November 2026

47664964R00029